T0197300

Sex

Rekindling Your Passion

Is

with a Hot Break

Love

SEAN MOORE

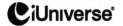

SEX IS LOVE
REKINDLING YOUR PASSION WITH A HOT BREAK

iUniverse books may be ordered through booksellers or by contacting:

iUniverse
1663 Liberty Drive
Bloomington, IN 47403
www.iuniverse.com
1-800-Authors (1-800-288-4677)

ISBN: 978-1-5320-5934-6 (sc)
ISBN: 978-1-5320-5933-9 (e)

Library of Congress Control Number: 2018912936

Print information available on the last page.

iUniverse rev. date: 10/29/2018

PREFACE

The matters of sex are no longer taboo. Even though the human race took hundreds of years to reach this point, we now have the freedom to discuss everything about sex. Since sex is the most basic and powerful motivating energy of life, it's good to explore untried possibilities and tap into the full potential of sexuality to enrich relationships between men and women.

This book has nothing to do with the negative side of sexuality, such as the sex trade, pornography, and sexual abuse. The sole intention here is to encourage people to achieve as much goodness from sex as possible, based on the belief that doing so is indisputably the right thing. Most everything has a good side and a bad side; that's the way things are in nature. There will always be people who try to exploit good things, including sexuality, for their own selfish motives. For now, however, the negative side of sexuality is not our concern. Instead, let's pursue the unmatchable happiness of sex.

The freedom of expression that we enjoy today, which has been hard earned, has revealed a path to detailed knowledge about the secrets of sex. Through that process, embarrassment about sex has largely been eliminated, but has this change really improved the quality of male-female relationships? No, most people have gained little from this newly developed understanding of sexuality. Even now, they just act on their basic urge for sex, enjoying it but missing out on a world of possibility.

It's time to closely examine this issue. As we look at the world around us, human sexuality isn't doing so well. We see unhappy marriages and a climbing divorce rate, no improvement in the incidence of reported sexual abuse, and an increase in serious sex crimes. We need a fresh affirmation of the goodness of sex, so that people will stop thinking of sexual enjoyment as just a side benefit of procreation. There is much more to sexuality that can help make male-female relationships amazingly enjoyable.

Sex is abundantly present these days, everywhere and in everything, but in most cases we're simply exploiting the superficial excitement associated with the idea of sex rather than tapping into the real goodness of sex. After talking with many people about relationships and sex, I have the feeling that society has became more selfish and uncaring. Focused on momentary gratification, people are not willing to take even short-term responsibility to learn about one another's physical and emotional needs. This skulking away from responsibility could be based on shyness or embarrassment about going into the details of physical and emotional aspects of relationships.

We do a lot of talking about sex, but few people make a sincere attempt to enjoy the positive possibilities of sex and use it specifically to improve and deepen their relationships. There's a lot of information available to help eliminate the embarrassment of talking about sex, but little help in removing embarrassment about the sexual act itself. We need a more detailed, bolder, and deeper understanding of human sexuality. In male-female relationships, an emphasis on the importance of sex can be interesting, meaningful, and realistic, since sex is an extremely intimate bonding experience. The emotional side of relationships can involve other issues, but good sex is the best way to achieve and maintain a rewarding male-female relationship.

This book is based on my own real-life experiences, insights gained from numerous other people's experiences, and long years of thinking and planning. Many people, including some of my closest friends, have willingly revealed to me their most personal sexual experiences, which has helped make this book more accurate and interesting, I thank them here from the bottom of my heart.

My motivation for writing this book has been to demonstrate that there is much to explore and enjoy about positive sex. I've tried to use my experiences of good sexuality to generate creative ideas and realistic approaches that can be effective in real life. If this book shows people how to be happier through good sex and helps them discover new aspects, dimensions, and possibilities for positive sex, then I've accomplished my task.

I truly believe that readers who sincerely try to understand and employ the core ideas of this book will enjoy amazing experiences of positive sex. This book also offers a valuable asset for men and women who are looking for more meaningful, wonderfully enjoyable relationships. I passionately hope that every adult will reach the peak of love through reinventing sex. Sex is love, and this book can help you go on the happiest roller-coaster ride imaginable.

Thank you.

Sincerely,
Sean Moore

This book is dedicated to women and men in relationships who want to experience a distinctive dimension of love through a complete act of sex.

Contents

One

Sex?

What is sex? From a physiological perspective, it's about X and Y chromosomes, body changes at puberty, the differences between male and female genital organs, and so on. Sexuality is relatively simple if we aren't seeking an in-depth understanding of it. If we sincerely want to understand what sexuality really is, however, it's not that simple.

The basic purpose, as nature intended it, of sex between a man and a woman is simply the continuation of our species. Our life journey begins from a woman's vagina, and as newborn babies, we are first identified by our sexuality. When the news of a child's birth is announced, the first question is typically, "Is it a boy or a girl?" Everything begins with sex. Nature's male-female organizational structure is far more amazing than most of us realize, but are we deriving as much good out of it as possible?

At the age of three or four, boys and girls start to notice and become curious about the difference in what's between their legs. That difference usually leads to an intense mutual attraction between male and female adolescents, even though they might not understand its original purpose. When boys and girls become adults, most begin to yearn for a personal close friend and partner from the opposite sex. Typically boys want girlfriends and girls want boyfriends to satisfy their inescapable sexual urges. This strong sexual magnetism prevails everywhere in the lives of men and women, resulting in many childbirths and some happiness. Although this truth has never been fully exposed, there are many more dimensions to sexuality that both sexes can explore, if we are ready to go for it and be happily surprised by those experiences.

The sexual urge is almost totally irresistible and inescapable. Most people are used to the manipulations of this extreme force, whether they have some knowledge of how it works or they're totally ignorant of sex's strange ways. If you want to know the power of the sexual urge, ask someone who practices celibacy for religious or other reasons. They'll tell you how hard it is to endure and ignore the pressure of sexual manifestations in the body. Nature actually lures young men and women into indulging in sexual activity for the purpose of childbirth. The continuation of our species isn't a result of everyone engaging in sexual activity as a duty or responsibility; instead, we are naturally seduced by the amazing power of the sexual urge.

What makes this sexual urge so extremely irresistible? The answer to that question is a secret— and yet not a secret. It's the thrilling physical intensity and emotional enjoyment of the sexual act. The happiness of sex is hard to define, but it is truly real and there's nothing to match it.

Here's another perspective. Just imagine that one day, for whatever reason, women stop having babies. Everything in this world would lose its sense of purpose and meaning, because there would be nothing to hope for in the future. Actually, sex is the first step in the process that gives life its meaning. When a man and woman fall in love and have sex, attracted by the magnetism of its intense enjoyment, and later have a child, it gives purpose and meaning to their lives.

The fact that sex gives life its meaning is indisputable. Our goal in this book is to find sensible, effective ways to use the intense happiness generated by sex to uplift male-female relationships and make them more meaningful and lasting.

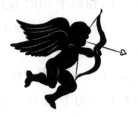

Euphoria

I n reality, how much happiness is involved in sex and how intense is sexual pleasure? The excitement and pleasure of the sexual act is life's most intense experience for all human beings—and probably for all living creatures. It's a fact that having sex is the most extreme physical experience and the most significant emotional experience for human adults. That's because nature has to lure us into having sex to make sure that our species continues, as discussed in the previous chapter.

If we tried to decide on the most exciting experience that's possible in life, a few ideas would come up. Being the powerful ruler of a nation, accepted and revered by all, or a successful businessperson would be exciting. Likewise, there must be great satisfaction in being an actor, musician, or writer who is loved by millions. But the good feelings that come from being powerful, rich, and famous are always tangled up with other people and things, and they tend to involve unexpected ups and downs. This is also true for people who like adventure and thrills—climbing a tall mountain, free-falling from an airplane, travelling around the world in a yacht, riding the world's tallest roller coaster, and so on. Such thrilling adventures often involve great struggle, expense, and risk, and most of the time the results aren't worth the effort.

Even though people enjoy the excitement of being powerful, successful, rich, famous, and adventurous, it's an indisputable fact that most of us wouldn't be willing to give up sexual pleasures in return for those big experiences. Sexual pleasure holds a unique place in our lives that cannot be replaced by any other experience. If forced to choose between sexual pleasures and being rich and famous, most of us would choose the former. In fact, being powerful, rich, or famous usually increases our expectations about the possibilities for achieving greater sexual pleasure; that's just how this world and human behavior work.

All the riches and fame in the world aren't an acceptable substitute for sexual pleasures, especially for men.

Since sexual pleasure is the most intense and exciting form of pleasure available for human beings, let's examine a few basic requirements for achieving sexual pleasure. If a man and a woman can come together in their most basic form, which is their naked bodies, with open minds, positive attitudes, and no hidden motives, shedding all shyness and inhibitions, and wholeheartedly engage in sex, they will have an intense, wholesome, and pleasurable experience.

When sex happens, it doesn't matter how much money you have in your bank account. Material well-being can enhance the experience of sexual pleasure if it's used in a positive way, but anyone who thinks that material prosperity is the only way to achieve a better sexual experience is sadly mistaken.

Another interesting thing about sex is that when we try to decide on the most memorable events in our lives, several of them will probably involve good sexual experiences. The sheer happiness and highly enjoyable, intense, and pure effect on our wholeness makes sexual pleasure highly memorable. Sex is secretive and mystic, and sexual experience will stay with us for our whole lives because of the deep, sweet marks it leaves in our brains.

Every adult human being knows that the good feelings generated by sex are special and extremely interesting, whether they see it from a natural or a mystical perspective. But are we really using this abundant sexual pleasure to make our lives more enjoyable and to make male-female relationships more intimate and meaningful? When we truthfully consider the things happening all around us, for most of us the answer is probably no.

Three

Roadblocks to Eden

E veryone knows that an abundance of uniquely pleasurable sexual experience is available to any two naked adults whose minds aren't polluted by crooked intentions, but are we getting enough of this easily available pleasure? If not, we must look seriously for ways to enhance our lives through sexuality, because the wholesome experience of sexuality is definitely worth the effort. To attain long-lasting sexual happiness, however, we must identify and remove the obstacles that are blocking our path. Achieving that goal demands sincerity, a lot of patience, and a willingness to search deep inside our minds.

When passing through adolescence toward adulthood, every man and woman naturally becomes intensely aware that there are some mystically good things about genital organs. To our astonishment, it becomes clear that the genital organs have a strange ability to provide an extreme kind of enjoyment, and naturally we realize that to experience that intense good feeling, a woman needs a man and a man needs a woman.

In adolescence and early adulthood, we must overcome many obstacles to enjoy the happiness available through our sexual organs, but those obstacles have a meaningful purpose. Most of us live with our parents through our early twenties, inside their protective circle and within view of other elders, which is a big obstacle to freely enjoying sexual happiness in our younger years. Other obstacles include the warnings that we get from teachers and other school officials, our own fears and lack of knowledge about sex, and the difficulty of finding a secluded place and sufficient freedom to fulfill our sexual wishes. All of these obstacles to sexual enjoyment at a young age actually serve a positive purpose by giving us enough time to learn about all the good in sexuality and some bad things that can happen on the road to a sex life. In effect, these obstacles are preparing us for an enjoyable "sexploration." Young people should wait until they mature enough and have a good understanding about these things before they enter into a sincere relationship, so the obstacles mentioned here don't need to be removed.

However, the obstacles to a wholesome experience of sexual enjoyment in adult relationships are more difficult to deal with. Some are well known and might seem simple, but that doesn't mean they can be easily resolved. Many obstacles along the path to total sexual enjoyment, though vague and ambiguous, are quite real, and their removal requires hard work and determination. Wise and sincere actions, combined with sufficient patience, will help us achieve the goal of real sexual enjoyment to the maximum.

Money

The first obstacle to long-lasting sexual enjoyment might be a lack of sufficient money, though this is typically not a problem for younger men and women. The younger years are the purest phase in male-female relationships because facts cannot penetrate that romantic world. But later, when women and men enter into serious adult relationships, they will face many challenging realities for the first time, including a lack of money. In fact, an unsatisfactory material situation could be their biggest hurdle.

This financial sufficiency issue could affect the male-female relationship in many ways, obviously including their sexual enjoyment. Having a good life depends on having enough money—there's no doubt about that. But it isn't wise to allow financial insufficiency to override full enjoyment in relationships. Nevertheless, financial sufficiency is better because it allows partners to engage in sexual interaction in comfortable surroundings and a reasonably worry-free atmosphere. The possibility for a full celebration of sexuality is definitely enhanced by a nice house with heating and air-conditioning, cozy bedrooms furnished with comfortable beds, expensive sex toys, high-quality condoms, and other amenities.

In general, financial insufficiency is a real hurdle on the path to wholesome sexual enjoyment for many people. On the other hand, being rich doesn't guarantee a long-lasting, happy sex life. That requires a few other important things, in addition to money.

Other Family Members

In a serious male-female relationship, especially since it's one of the most important purposes of a relationship of this kind, children will be born without much delay, and that will change everything about the relationship forever, including sexual interactions.

Children are the most basic source of happiness and meaning in life, but they take a good chunk of their parents' privacy, time, and sometimes even peace of mind. All good things come at a price. Having enough privacy and time for sexual enjoyment is a serious issue for parents, and it gets even more problematic when children reach the age of four or five.

Another thing that can jeopardize a couple's private life is when other family members must live with them. Regardless of the reasons, if partners aren't getting enough of the most wonderful reward of male-female relationships, that can be truly disappointing. This issue of lack of sexual enjoyment must be seriously addressed, and the time and energy devoted to overcoming this issue will not be wasted.

Same Partner, Same Ways

Another important issue regarding sexual enjoyment for men and women, though interesting, can be a bit uncomfortable to discuss. In a committed relationship, the "same partner" half of the situation can't really be resolved. The "same ways" part isn't quite as simple to deal with, though it can be seen as a challenge and actually serve as a catalyst if the two partners seriously want to overcome it.

The "same ways" part of the issue is psychological, a matter of mind and behavior, invisible but real and hard to address. "Same partner, same ways" is a serious challenge in the journey toward long-lasting sexual enjoyment, but the good news is that we are capable of overcoming it with our superior intelligence. Any struggle for the most intense form of happiness available to us is absolutely worth the effort.

Sickness and Disability

There are challenges standing between us and all good things, and sexual enjoyment is no exception. Sickness and disability can be a serious obstruction to wholesome, happy, long-lasting sexual experience, because problems that affect our bodies will naturally affect our sex lives. Even though our focus here is specifically on sexuality, problems of the body can be multidimensional, sophisticated, and serious—well beyond the scope of this book.

Some sicknesses and disabilities can adversely affect sexual activities, such as erectile dysfunction, vulvodynia (vaginal pain), or vaginitis. These problems require earnest and prompt attention if we're serious about our sexual happiness and the overall health of our bodies for normal, happy living. Problems with sexual organs that diminish our sexual happiness might not affect our regular day-to-day life that much, but they will certainly destroy a large portion of our personal joy. Loss of sexual happiness is neither a small nor an unimportant matter. We should take any steps needed, as soon as possible, to restore our physical well-being even if the problem is related to our sexual organs and doesn't affect daily life. Life should be enjoyed to its fullest.

Age

Everything in life, the good and the bad, including our priceless sexual happiness, faces the certain and final attack of age. In other words, we're all getting older. People below the age of forty generally don't worry about getting old, nor should they. As we reach our midforties, however, getting old starts to become a reality, and we begin to feel the physical and psychological effects of aging.

As we get older, the bodily organs that lead us to the world of sexual bliss will also gradually begin to weaken. Unfortunately, many people are surprised, even shocked, by the first signs of getting old, which also affects their level of sexual activity. And many will almost immediately make the mistake of surrendering to the aging process, either consciously or unconsciously, because they're too lazy to fight for the sake of sexual happiness. Some people even hide their losing fight against aging from their partners, which is definitely not a wise approach.

Aging women tend to secretly give up the fight for sexual happiness sooner than men do. Most women will fiercely resist getting old externally, but they're more hesitant to keep up the secret internal fight and do the work needed to stay youthful and physically fit as long as possible. Therefore they lose the ability to immerse themselves in sexual happiness to the maximum attainable extent. But women should take serious steps to stay physically fit, because sexual happiness is more worthwhile than we generally realize. It's true that getting old is normal and unavoidable, but we don't have do it any sooner than necessary.

There may be other obstacles that did not get mentioned here, and plenty of totally unexpected variations of challenges can hinder our long-lasting enjoyment of sexual happiness. But any time and effort that we spend achieving the most intense good feeling of life is worthwhile.

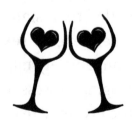

Men's Blocks

Unexpected enemies work from surprising places to prevent long-lasting sexual joy. Most of them come as external disturbances, but some work from inside the relationship itself, even without the knowledge of both partners.

Men and women are absolutely equal when it comes to the importance of the parts that we play and their relevance in fulfilling the wholeness of life. Until recent times, men were considered superior to women, and even in these modern days of open knowledge, religious zealots and other narrow-minded people want to keep it that way for their own selfish motives.

It's true that men generally have more physical strength than women, but looking at the situation from other specific perspectives, we could argue just the opposite. As discussed in a previous chapter, childbirth gives meaning to life, and yet the participation of men in that process basically ends with a relatively brief, though enjoyable, act of sex. After that, men more or less stay out of their partner's struggle to give birth, and in some cases they also assume little responsibility for taking care of the child as well. From this point of view, we could argue that the female gender holds the superior position in making life meaningful. Nevertheless, when we broadly consider all aspects of a shared life and do the math honestly, the equality of the two genders is confirmed—which is absolutely the wise and better path to choose.

Women and men are equal in a basic and general sense, but being equal doesn't mean that they aren't different. This is an important point, especially when it comes to issues of intimate male-female relationships and sexual enjoyment. Even regarding physical strength, it is better to view men as different than to consider them superior. The difference in physical strength between women and men is just one of many ways that nature balances the male and female genders to achieve full function in life. People used to joke that men are from Mars and women are from Venus. This is a bit of an exaggeration, because men and women are alike in many ways. In others ways, however, women and men are truly different, and that makes male-female relationships interesting in some positive respects.

The fact that men and women are different, though it makes sense on many levels, also creates some specific problems for both genders regarding long-lasting sexual enjoyment. When we explicitly examine the typical gender persona of men, some unexpected and compelling aspects become apparent, including an especially important one that needs to be addressed. To put it simply, men are naturally more selfish and self-centered than women. They tend to be less caring and more insensitive to the opposite sex, specifically when it comes to the matter of sexual enjoyment. Many men, especially in their younger years, talk about sexual encounters with women in terms of achievement or triumph. Men boast about making women surrender to them with a specific sex act or tricking women into submitting themselves for the sexual enjoyment of the man. This approach is obviously insensitive and self-centered.

Sexual joy should come from a mutual, equal quest to attain one of the greatest joys in life; it should have nothing to do with one person surrendering to or triumphing over someone else. I'm not using the words *selfish*, *self-centered*, and *insensitive* in the sense of evil psychopaths and criminals, but rather from the perspective of a serious issue that normal people often face regarding sexuality.

The selfishness, self-centeredness, or uncaring insensitivity of men doesn't necessarily come from evil intentions or a negative mind-set, but rather from a deep, primitive male instinct. The same instinct that drives every living organism to fight for survival pushes men to deposit their seeds in as many places as possible. This basic instinct sometimes subconsciously manifests as insensitive male behavior, which is the issue here. Regardless of the reason, this uncaring male behavior doesn't work well when men and women are seeking sexual happiness, whether in short- or long-term relationships.

Does this mean that all men are bad? No, not at all. Unfortunately some men are bad to various degrees, and this uncaring attitude or insensitivity is a reality for many men. It's present in all men at a minimal level, but when it's allowed to grow and exceed an acceptable level, it's definitely counterproductive for an enjoyable relationship and sexual happiness. Men should always be careful to be in control of this matter of selfish insensitivity. The human race has come a long way from our ancient beginnings, and it can be really disappointing that we're still in the grip of this primitive instinct.

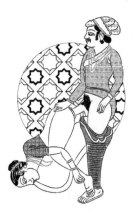

Women's Blocks

To get something really valuable and enjoyable out of life is truly a struggle. When it comes to the matter of fruitful and effective male-female relationships, that struggle might sometimes be invisible, but it's definitely complex. In maintaining a flourishing, long-lasting male-female sexual relationship, the differences in gender-based behaviors further complicate that struggle.

As is the case for men, women have a few blocks along the path to long-lasting, thriving sexual enjoyment. The most important block for many women is that having sex is not primarily about the enjoyment and thrill of the sex act itself, but for other benefits that are considered more important, serious, or meaningful. For many women, the goal of sex is to acquire a partner, get pregnant and have a baby, or make their male partner happy enough to stay in the relationship. In other words, many women don't engage in sex primarily for their personal sexual enjoyment. Most women are willing to be satisfied with only a secondhand kind of sexual experience, and they're missing out on the more wholesome, joyous experience of sex.

Of course, women go through a brief period of intense sexual fascination as young adults. But everything changes when girls enter their twenties and shift to using sexuality to achieve specific benefits. This use of sexuality is often actually a positive manifestation of the ancient female instinct to fulfill their natural duty by continuing the species and accepting responsibility for the care and well-being of offspring.

There's nothing wrong with wanting to have children or prioritizing our partner's happiness to achieve a long, happy relationship. In fact, there is an admirable aspect of self-sacrifice to some of those approaches. Nevertheless, when women minimize the importance of their own personal sexual joy in a relationship, that's a huge loss and a big mistake in the greater experience of life.

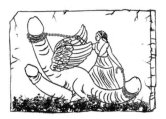

Dealing with Blocks

I f it's important enough that a problem be solved, then we will surely find ways to solve it. Sometimes just changing our perspective will reveal that a problem isn't really hard to solve or perhaps that it isn't actually a problem at all.

When it comes to sexual enjoyment, generally people present ideas only about such things as how to properly perform foreplay, talk dirty better, and overcome premature ejaculation, or about the most enjoyable sex positions, multiple orgasms, and so on. The kind of issues discussed in this chapter are usually avoided in sex manuals. Perhaps there is the assumption that these issues are outside the context of sexual enjoyment or the belief that these issues must be dealt with separately because they're too delicate and/or offensive to some people. But the reality is that these are the core issues preventing partners from enjoying a thrilling sex life, so we should discuss these matters openly.

Dealing with Money Matters

Material sufficiency, or having enough money for a comfortable life, is indisputably the most important and basic thing that people need. For people living in hostile situations and struggling to satisfy their most basic needs, issues concerning sexual enjoyment will not be at the top of their priority list.

Our planet's population today can be divided into three general living conditions. The vast majority of people don't earn enough money to provide anything more than their basic needs for survival. A small percentage of the population makes enough money to live debt-free with needed comforts. The third group, a minuscule number of people, have far more money than they need and have all necessary comforts plus unnecessary luxuries.

Having enough wealth is good, and there's nothing wrong with having more than enough. Material affluence can work as a catalyst to increase the quality of sexual experiences in relationships, but only if used wisely. An abundance of material comforts doesn't guarantee a really happy sex life, because male-female relationships must be nurtured and maintained on their own terms.

People who have an adequate—or more than adequate—level of material wealth cannot blame money if they are experiencing a lack of wholeness in their relationships or diminished quality in their sexual enjoyment. People who aren't earning enough money to live comfortably can, to some extent, blame material insufficiency for their inability to achieve sexual enjoyment, but they must remember that an abundance of wealth doesn't guarantee that anyone will experience the joy of sexuality in its fullness.

Since material abundance is not the deciding factor in who does or does not achieve real sexual happiness, that means that people who are struggling with financial insufficiency nevertheless can hope to find other paths to the bliss of sexuality. People who don't have enough will keep trying to attain financial sufficiency; that's a basic human behavior, but it may take more time than they expect. Meanwhile, blaming material insufficiency for sexual unhappiness is a huge waste of precious, limited time that we can never get back. Sexual enjoyment is a time-sensitive matter, and it's never a good idea to wait until we acquire all of our desired comforts before focusing on true sexual happiness.

Let your day job and other troubles of life go their normal, ordinary way, at the same time that your relationship travels down its private, vibrant, romantic path of love. Couples who want to be happy must accept this approach wholeheartedly and practice it with total determination. A companionship that is unaffected by the disturbances of life around it will last for a long time, and the sexual happiness in that relationship will be unusually strong. This ideal relationship will never disappoint even though it has some shortcomings, but a relationship without sexual enjoyment is certain to disappoint.

Sexual happiness can also dissolve the day-to-day stress of life, especially that which results from the fight to attain material affluence. Since this approach will surely ease the daily hardships of life, it is absolutely a win-win situation.

In a nutshell, let money matters go their own way while the joy of your relationship strides on down its private path, and exploit the extreme pleasures of male-female companionship to ease the stress of attaining material affluence. Making a sincere attempt to achieve your goals is what matters.

Dealing with Other Family Members

There are some problems that we simply cannot get rid of completely, so the only thing to do is adapt to those problems and happily live with them. Sometimes sharing a home with other family members can make it difficult for a couple to engage in sexual interaction at a normal frequency. Obviously we cannot get rid of other family members for any reason, so this can be a delicate issue to deal with. From an unbiased and truly sincere point of view, this can be a significant issue for couples trying to have a wholesome, enjoyable sex life. The best way to deal with this problem is to confront the situation honestly and find solutions strictly within the secret private world of each couple.

One thing couples can do is be flexible and take advantage of any opportunity for intimacy, rather than adamantly sticking with usual practices. Always be ready, day or night, for a delightful sexual experience, whether in your bedroom or in a washroom, closet, or basement. This doesn't mean that couples living with other family members should always be thinking, *How, where, and when can we have sex?* But when other family members aren't at home or in a couple's private spaces, we shouldn't miss those opportunities for sexual bliss for the sake of relationships. Sometimes this just takes shrewd intelligence and a bit of an unorthodox approach. Sexual encounters in the midst of unusual circumstances can be unexpectedly thrilling experiences. For example, a quickie—a brief sexual encounter—can be extremely satisfying and become a precious lifetime memory.

Any couple who really wants to keep up the bliss of their companionship through sex will find ways to make that happen, if they sincerely work on doing so.

Dealing with the Same Partner, Same Ways

In a committed male-female relationship, surprisingly few sexual issues arise that are unusual or even unacceptable, but there are a few. The "same partner, same ways" issue is one of them. Part of the delicate nature of this particular issue is that it doesn't make sense to view "same partner" as a problem in a committed relationship. It's also true that the "ways" of a sexual relationship tend to remain static simply because the partners are always the same.

Fortunately, this is not an unsolvable problem. People are sufficiently intelligent to learn new behaviors with which to supplement or replace old ones. Regarding sexual practices, the key is a clear willingness to take serious action and a determination to maintain the passion of the relationship.

When couples decide to overcome the problem of "same partner, same ways," they can make changes in two basic ways. First, have sex only while using new positions. Put away your overused positions, at least until the new ones become humdrum, and avoid using the basic missionary position forever—or at least for a long time. Attempting new positions will definitely add unexpected thrills and enjoyment to a couple's sex life.

The other basic strategy for changing the "same ways" of sex play is to abandon the place where you're accustomed to having sex—the same bedroom, the same bed, and so on. Don't have sex in that same old place, at least for a while, but think of it as just one among many places in the house where you can have sex. Take your erotic games to a couch, a chair, a kitchen counter, the dining room table, or even the laundry room. Also try having sex in small spaces, such as a small washroom, the back seat of your car, or even leaning against the car inside your closed garage. As long as you're in a safe, private place, letting your imaginations go wild is a great way to rejuvenate your relationship and put you back on the path to a long-lasting, enjoyable sex life.

Dealing with Sickness and Disability

Unfortunately life is not always fair, and some people have to live with some kind of illness or permanent disability. It's not within the scope of this book to propose a definitive, totally satisfactory resolution to the challenges faced by those people as they seek sexual enjoyment. Also, it obviously would not be appropriate for us to approach sickness and disability primarily from the perspective of sexual enjoyment.

However, we can explore useful ideas to manage physical challenges that have a direct, negative effect on a couple's sex life, such as impotency, erectile dysfunction, vaginal dryness, vaginal pain, and venereal disease. Such ailments can be treated and, to a surprising extent, cured with disciplined, determined effort on the part of the sufferer. The most important thing is simply to be willing to see a qualified doctor. Any couple who really knows what they're missing out on, in the absence of happy sexual interactions, will surely take this first step to bring the joy of sexuality into their lives. In particular, anyone suffering from a venereal disease should take action immediately.

Dealing with Matters of Age

Don't even think about getting old until you actually do. In fact, it's best just to imagine that you will never be old. Everything and everyone is continuously getting older. Aging is inevitable, but worrying about it is pointless. To avoid missing out on the precious joy of sex, we must live in the present, completely apart from worries about the future. We can worry about, plan for, and work toward lots of other things, but sexual happiness is all about immersing ourselves in the present.

In a good relationship, partners will be enthusiastically active in their sex life without allowing many gaps. If we're having long erotically inactive gaps, we should remind ourselves that time is passing and we're missing out on the most special kind of happiness. Also, if couples don't stay present in their sex lives as long as they can, the effects of aging will start to show up a bit early. Yes, of course, everyone will get old someday, and visible signs of aging will start to appear around the age of fifty. But that doesn't mean that life is almost over—the truth is that there's a lot more life still to enjoy.

As discussed earlier, as we get old erectile dysfunction, vaginal pain and dryness, and other physical problems can hinder our celebration of sex. Couples must do everything possible to alleviate those problems, such as taking advantage of all available medical and psychological treatments and making necessary lifestyle changes—regular exercise, healthful eating, and so on. The thrill and happiness of sex is too much of a good thing to lose. Too many people think of themselves as getting old earlier than they should. Defying age can be a fight against nature, but in this case it's definitely worth it.

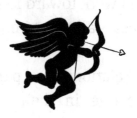

Seven

Dealing with Women's Blocks

As mentioned earlier, most women engage in sex not primarily for the thrill or happiness of the sex act itself, but instead to make sure that they have a few basic things needed for their existence. This might not be true for every woman, but it is true for many. Those women might not even be consciously aware of their motivation, which makes them unable to enjoy their sexuality in all its richness.

Women of all ages should search their own thoughts to find out what is true for them. When a woman realizes that she is engaging in sex only to maintain her relationship and to fulfill her duty regarding the continuation of our species, she should try to understand what she's actually missing out on. For a sincere and responsible person who isn't experiencing the pure happiness of sexuality, which is also a source of joy in our personal well-being, this is obviously not a small loss. Women in this situation should change their approach and learn to enjoy their sexuality solely because of the unique happiness that it brings, rather than for any other reasons.

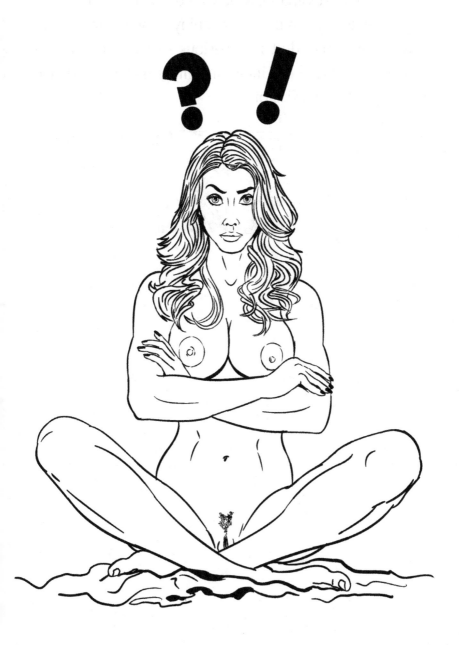

Efforts to overcome whatever obstacles are faced on the way to total, pure sexual enjoyment are absolutely worth it. Any adult in a serious relationship should live life to its fullest, including enjoying an abundance of the extreme bliss of sex.

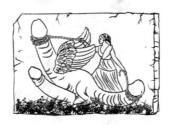

Chapter

Eight

Dealing with Men's Blocks

As discussed earlier, one of the most important issues that keep many people from enjoying the rich, multidimensional pleasures of sex is almost exclusive to men. The most basic motivation of an adult man for having a sexual relationship with an adult woman is to release sexual tension in the most satisfying way possible. This is a matter of basic instinct, and it leads many men to be self-centered, giving insufficient care and respect to the opposite sex. Whether they are aware of what they're doing or simply acting from base instinct, it is simply wrong of men to treat women only as a mechanism to satisfy their sexual cravings—or to treat them with anything less than respect and compassion in all aspects of the relationship.

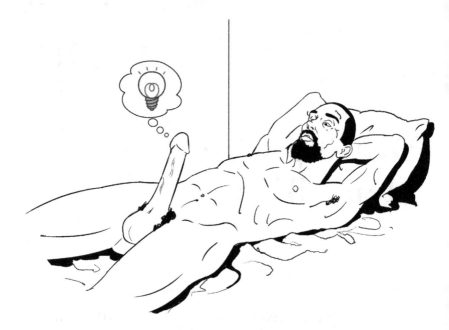

Some may argue that a man can hide his actual, hidden motivation and avoid hurting his partner's feelings by behaving politely and pleasantly. Yes, that might work for a while, but eventually a man's internal thoughts and emotions will be reflected in his external behavior, and then the woman will begin to sense that something is wrong. This dishonest approach on the man's part is not compatible with a rich, healthy, long-term relationship, so embracing a straightforward, positive approach will be more effective.

For a man who wants to pursue the goal of appropriate sexual behavior toward women, two simple strategies will quickly improve his attitude toward women and perhaps even eliminate the problem altogether. First, he should just imagine how he would feel if someone acted as though it was okay to exploit him just to achieve their own selfish goals. Obviously nobody appreciates being treated that way, so we shouldn't behave that way toward others. It's a simple fact that men should never approach women with a hidden intention of exploiting them to satisfy men's own selfish sexual craving. Imagining what it feels like to stand in another person's shoes is a simple but effective technique for understanding appropriate interpersonal behavior. A man who wants to maintain an enjoyable companionship with a woman must learn to think as though he's standing in her shoes.

The second strategy for insensitive men is an extension of the first one. Simply imagine how you would feel if someone approached your mother, sister, or daughter in an uncaring way for their own selfish motives. Absolutely nobody would feel good about that. When men interact with women, whether publicly or in private, they must always remember that every woman is somebody else's daughter, sister, or mother—and that they are all equally deserving of respect and compassion.

Again, I want to emphasize that not all men are insensitive or uncaring, just as some women aren't necessarily caring and selfless. However, anyone who practices these two basic strategies will surely see a positive change in their behavior toward others. The basic habit of treating others as you want to be treated can apply to everything in this world, and it will work magic in male-female relationships and lead to deeper sexual joy.

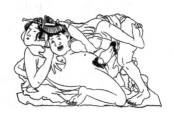

What A Wonderful Sex!

E very adult has the basic, natural instinct that by engaging in sex, they can experience a marvelous sort of happiness. As intelligent creatures, however, humans are driven to a deeper understanding of ourselves and the world around us, rather than relying simply on basic natural feelings. Trying to learn as much as we can about our sexuality will reveal how much more goodness it can deliver than we normally expect.

Even people who are well educated about the mysteriously vibrant possibilities of sexuality can go through times, after the heat of horniness cools down a bit, when the woman isn't wet enough or the man's erection isn't hard enough. This can happen to adults of any age, and although the causes for such disappointments might be minor, their effects will often be significant. These occasional lacks of libido, rather than resulting from some physical decline, might be indications that the time has come to reinvent and reconfirm the goodness of sexuality. Sexuality has huge potential to make our lives happier and even more thrilling, so our determined efforts to know more about it are definitely good.

The Best Good Feeling

Happiness is a fundamental goal of life, and one thing that can create intense good feelings in us is the act of sex. There is actually a scientific basis for the uniquely positive feeling that results from having sex. During intercourse, the brain secretes the hormone Oxytocin, also known as the happy hormone, hug hormone, cuddle chemical, moral molecule, or bliss hormone. These names reflect the variety of effects that oxytocin has on human behavior, in direct contrast to the effects produced by cortisol, the stress hormone.

So one way to guarantee that we'll generally enjoy life is to engage in sexual intercourse as often as we can, thus flooding our bodies with more and more oxytocin. Why waste a lot of time building up unrealistic expectations about life and chasing goals that have uncertain rewards? The good feeling that sex can deliver is sure and real, and this fact is strongly supported by scientific evidence.

In many situations, experiences that produce really good feelings are expensive, and we might not be able to share those experiences with anyone else. But when a woman and man in good companionship simply engage in sex, they share and help each other experience the intensely good feeling. Just have a lot of sex, produce more oxytocin, and be happier.

Strengthen Your Shield

Every second of our lives, we're surrounded by things that can make us sick—deadly viruses, bacteria, dust filled with allergen particles, and so on. Germs and other bad things are constantly trying to enter our body and make us ill, but we're protected by a built-in immune system that works to shield us from disease. The stronger our shield of immunity, the better, so we must do our part by maintaining a healthy lifestyle.

In recent years, numerous medical research studies conducted at highly reputed universities have clearly proven that sexual activity has positive effects on the human immune system. When people engage in sexual intercourse, their level of the antibody Immunoglobulin (IgA) increases to well above normal. Immunoglobulin boosts the effectiveness of the human immune system and offers extra protection against cold, flu, and other ailments. The studies also demonstrate that people who engage in sexual intercourse more than twice a week will benefit even more.

In many situations, achieving good and worthwhile results requires us to endure long hours of boring, hard work. But when men and women engage in wild sex—an extremely enjoyable activity that is sensuously interesting, encouraging, and meaningful—their immune systems become stronger and stronger. Maintaining a stronger shield of immunity by engaging in sex more often is undoubtedly a wise thing to do. Be more sexually active and make your immune system stronger.

Young Radiance

Here's some good news for all men and women. When we frequently engage in sex, surreal and totally unexpected good things can happen. Following a wholesome session of sexual intercourse, people sometimes feel like they have a youthful glow, and recent medical research studies indicate that this is true.

At the time of sexual activity, especially during and immediately after intercourse, production of the hormones Testosterone and Estrogen dramatically increases. This increased presence of testosterone in men and estrogen in women slows down the body's aging process and gives a radiance to skin. People who regularly enjoy wholesome sexual intercourse, as opposed to those who infrequently engage in sex just to relieve tension, can reverse time's effect on their bodies with an extra glow to their skin. Some research studies have shown that people who enjoy sex more frequently look even twelve years younger than sexually lazy people.

So there's no point in wasting time and money on painstaking treatments and bitter medicines to escape aging. Staying busy with the extreme pleasure of wild sex is the best thing women and men can do. Immerse yourself in wholesome sexual intercourse and stay young as long as you can.

The Most Enjoyable Exercise

We are surrounded today by a growing awareness of the benefits of healthful eating and physical fitness, including meticulously planned workouts involving various forms of exercise. Many people are desperately anxious to keep their bodies in good shape so that they can enjoy life more and live longer. To achieve that goal, people spend a lot of money and endure harsh workouts, although they might feel bitter about having to do so.

Almost every day, a new fitness guru emerges on the Internet or television with a new exercise plan that claims to be far more effective than previous ones. Fitness-frenzied people will chase these phony experts with money, even though they might have been deceived many times before. In the midst of all this physical fitness buzz and health-related stress, people seem unaware of an exciting and enjoyable workout that also efficiently burns calories.

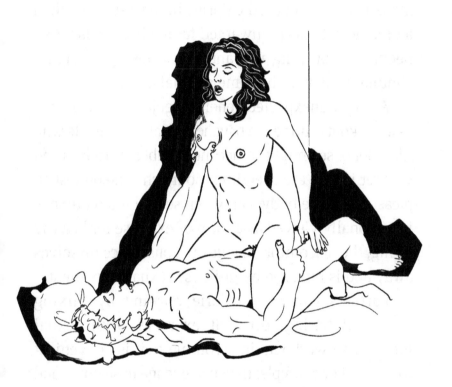

Staying fit is all about burning away extra calories and not accumulating fat. When adults engage in sex play, they burn an average of five calories per minute, so an hour of wholesome sexual celebration will burn away three hundred calories per person. If an adult engages in sex games every other day, they'll burn almost fifteen hundred calories in ten days, which is a great way to keep unwanted fat in check. Also, two people are burning unwanted calories by engaging simultaneously in the same sensual exercise.

Another unexpected benefit of enjoying a lot of sex as a workout routine is a psychological one. People who like a lot of sex might sometimes doubt themselves and wonder if they are spending too much time on lustful pleasures of the body. But when sexual intercourse is intentionally viewed as a form of exercise for healthy living, the discomfort of a guilty conscience dissolves away and is replaced by guiltless sexual enjoyment.

Partners can plan calorie burning by mixing the usual boring, difficult exercises with sexual intercourse workouts in a routine that is convenient for them. For example, they can engage in sex play and more conventional workouts on alternate weekdays, or three days per week can be spent on "sexercise" and the other four days on regular exercises. With a careful healthful eating practice, a couple could even totally avoid the usual boring exercises and adapt to engaging in sexual celebrations as their only form of exercise.

The bottom line is that we can immerse ourselves in more frequent sexual intercourse as a guiltless pleasure and live longer in a healthier body.

Do Good to Your Heart

More and more encouraging facts about sex are being revealed these days, making the secret personal world of couples even more exciting. For example, recent studies have shown that when men and women involve in sexual intercourse, their blood pressure drops. Having at least two robust sessions of sexual intercourse per week will reduce the risk of heart disease by 50 percent in men and almost that much in women. Sexual activity, particularly sexual intercourse between men and women, has many positive effects on the physiological activity of the body by maintaining healthy balances of estrogen and testosterone, which is important for a healthy heart and arteries and avoiding heart-related risks.

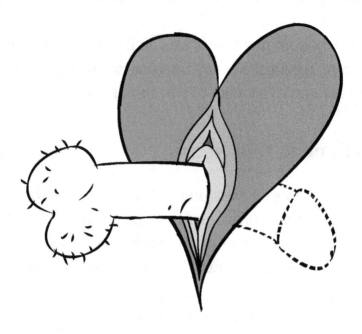

When we can indulge in an activity, such as sexual intercourse, that's interesting, exciting, and has such a good effect on our physical and psychological well-being, is there any point in being sexually lazy or avoiding sex altogether? This is just one more good reason for having more sex.

Amazing Painkiller

The next time you experience pain in your back, shoulder, hip, or knee, or the next time you're afflicted by a mild headache or even a migraine, don't rush for a remedy that contains artificial chemicals. Instead, pause and try a promising cure that's completely natural and extremely enjoyable. When pain attacks, invite your adult partner to have sexual intercourse for the relief of that pain. This isn't just wishful thinking or an old wives' tale; serious research studies have proven that sexual intercourse relieves pain.

The natural chemicals and hormones, especially endorphins, produced by the human body while engaged in sexual intercourse to the point of orgasm deliver potent pain relief. Many women who participated in those research studies revealed that even masturbation noticeably reduces various kinds of body pains, including headaches. This is just one more meaningful reason to indulge more in the pleasures of sex.

Sound Sleep

The importance of sleep does not need to be explained. Anyone who has been awake for just sixteen hours will long to lie down and go to sleep. Somehow a few hours of sound sleep can feel like a brief visit to heaven. We need sleep to stay healthy, but these days many people aren't enjoying enough good sleep. Many people don't understand that a lack of sleep is causing them to be ill. Even when they learn about the nasty effects of sleep deprivation, people tend to depend on unproven remedies and artificial medicines with unsatisfying partial results.

The good news, supported by numerous research studies, is that one of the positive effects of sexual activity is good sleep. Sexual intercourse and orgasm produce the hormones Prolactin and Oxytocin, which are capable of inducing deep sleep in both men and women. It's amazing that women and men can come together and indulge in lovemaking, with the extra benefit of a good night's sleep. Even masturbation will do the trick and help you sleep better.

One suggestion is that couples have sex on weeknights, sleep soundly, and be energized for work the next morning. On Saturday and Sunday, having morning sex and staying in bed longer is a good way to enjoy the weekend. Couples who don't have a typical workweek can set a sex-and-sleep schedule suitable to their lifestyle. Enjoy more sex, sleep well, and live a long, healthy life.

Effective Stress Relief

We cannot escape the residual stress of day-to-day life. An accumulation of mental and/or psychological fatigue is unhealthy and will seriously disrupt normal life in unforeseeable ways. Before we reach a breaking point, we need to relieve our stress so that we can lead a balanced and enjoyable life. Even our thoughts naturally affect the physiological chemistry of our bodies. That's why erotic fantasies cause women's vaginas to get wet and men to get erections and pre-ejaculate.

Avoiding stressful situations isn't a realistically workable solution. Getting rid of stress requires that our bodies produce enough good, stress-fighting chemicals. Some medications, made of artificial chemicals, relieve stress in extreme situations, but obviously that's not a healthy option. A good way to fight stress is to stimulate the body to secrete good hormones by doing things such as relaxing in beautiful places, listening to nice music, or enjoying many other forms of art.

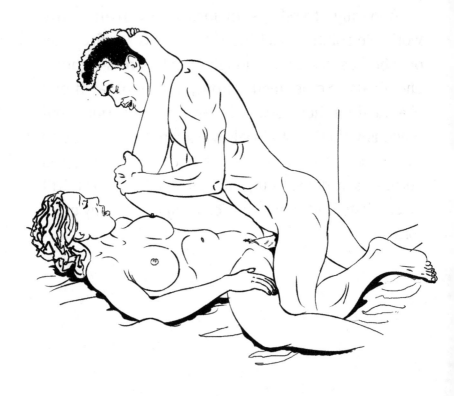

One of the best ways for adults to make lots of stress-reducing hormones is to engage as often as possible in wild sex. During sex play, our bodies busily secrete oxytocin and other good hormones that wash away stress like magic. What a great bonus!

Lighter Menses and Better Bladder Control

One important matter that makes women different from men is menses, the monthly period. This is nature's process of producing an egg every twenty-eight days to be fertilized by male sperm and grow into a new life. For many women the menses period, which lasts about five days a month, can be quite uncomfortable and even painful.

Research studies conducted on the subject of human sexuality have clearly demonstrated that women who have sexual intercourse or masturbate at least two or three times a week experience lighter menses complications. Although it's amusing to think of resolving one of the hardships of sexuality through sexual activity, it's also good news that sexual engagement can help women tackle the problems associated with their monthly period.

Another useful finding of research studies is that frequent sexual intercourse that concludes in intense orgasms results in better bladder control, especially for women. Thirty to thirty-five percent of women, mostly after middle age, experience some degree of incontinence as their pelvic base muscles lose strength and their ability to control urination deteriorates. During orgasm, strong waves of contractions occur in the pelvic base muscles, strengthening these muscles much like Kegel exercises do. Stronger muscles provide better bladder control and reduce urine leakage issues—yet another reason to immerse yourself in sexual intercourse as often as possible.

Good News for Prostate

The special fluid produced by the male prostate gland nourishes and carries sperm to the grand finale fireworks of every sexual encounter. At the height of orgasm, contractions in the prostate gland shoot semen deep into the woman's vagina. Those are the moments of which every adult male dreams. Although all aspects of sexuality, including prostate glands, fall within a romantic aura of intense and exciting experience for adults, sometimes we also have to face some uncomfortable realities. Prostate cancer is one of those realities.

Approximately one in eight men contracts prostate cancer. One research study on the subject of male sexuality revealed an interesting statistic: men who ejaculate more than twenty times a month are less likely to develop prostate cancer. It could be that one result of frequent ejaculations is that the prostate gland system get freshened regularly, which decreases the chances of developing cancer or other illnesses. Any body part that gets proper exercise and regular use will naturally stay healthy longer. Any accumulation of fluids, including semen, inside the body for long periods of time is bad for us, so an occasional flushing out should be done for better health.

To ejaculate more than twenty times a month might not be a realistic possibility for most men, but at least twelve to fifteen times is also beneficial, and ejaculation by masturbation has the same positive effect as by sexual intercourse. Men should expel their "love juice" as frequently as possible without pushing them to exhaustion. Sex is extremely enjoyable, and since it can help to prevent disease, engaging in it frequently is obviously the best logical choice. Men, don't skip a chance for sex, and women, enjoy sex more often for your partner's health.

Libido Alert

Because the sexual urge is the basic driving force of life, it goes without saying that the libido, which is the mental energy that keeps the sexual urge alive and burning, is very important. The sexual urge is a physical drive for the release of sexual tension, but the libido is the passionate psychological desire to have sex. There can be several psychological, circumstantial, or physical reasons for a lack of libido, which can affect an adult's enthusiasm in all areas of life. Moving through life without much forward drive can be an uncomfortable burden, although searching for the reasons for sexual sluggishness can be quite puzzling.

The best way to fight a lack of enthusiasm is to boost the libido, and research studies on sexual behavior have shown that the best way to do that is to use the little libido that you have. It is like jump-starting a battery to start your car and then driving the car around to fully recharge the battery and make the car run more efficiently. Research studies have shown that having sex increases the desire for more sex; in other words, having sex heightens the libido and thus makes the body more capable of enjoying the intense experience of sexual happiness in abundance.

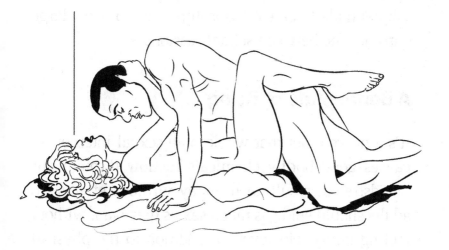

Sexual acts naturally stimulate the male body to produce more testosterone, and a strong testosterone presence in the bloodstream gives men more virility. Engaging in sexual intercourse makes women's vaginal muscles more flexible and creates increased lubrication and blood flow in the vaginal area. The result is that both men and women feel encouraged to engage in sex more often and they find sex more satisfying, which in turn makes life itself more enjoyable. The key to a vibrant male-female relationship is not to allow large gaps of time between sexual sessions.

A Better State of Being

It's a proven fact that wholesome sexual intercourse causes good bodily chemicals to flow through our bloodstream, resulting in many virtuous effects, so adults should enjoy as much sex as they want without feeling guilty. However, in addition to the physical benefits, sexual activity delivers many psychological benefits. Understanding those psychological effects will encourage more people to immerse themselves in sex play without any hesitation.

The urge to engage in sex is driven by a strong natural anticipation of an intensely positive experience. Adults spontaneously rationalize their desire for sex by thinking that they should engage in sex because they deserve to do so. Working together, these psychological aspects of sex impart a special feeling of achievement that elevates the person's self-esteem and adds to their overall sense of well-being.

Another fascinating aspect of sexual intercourse is the level of intimacy that it encourages in a relationship. Two adults come together and willingly reveal their naked bodies to each other, as though symbolically they have nothing to hide, and then part of one person's body enters the body of the other person and they become like a single organism. Only in a sexual relationship can two humans experience this extreme degree of intimacy. If love and a sincere, passionate caring for each other is also present, the relationship will thrive and make life worth living. It might not be easy to bring all these good things together, but it can be if the two partners truly love each other.

Glowing self-esteem, fueled by love and extraordinary sexual intimacy, will create a cozy sense of long-term well-being in a male-female relationship. For people who long for seasons of warm, lifelong happiness, immersing in frequent sessions of wholesome sexual intercourse is the most promising path to follow.

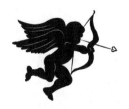

The Idea

For almost every adult, sexuality is a dream world filled with unique, wonderful experiences. Scientific research has proven that sexual acts have many positive effects on our bodies and minds, which is encouraging and exciting. Indulgence in sexual intercourse is intense and immensely satisfying—a great joy, dreamy and romantic. All these things are true, but is this the whole reality?

In everyday life, matters of sexuality might not always be so sweet and romantic. The dream world of sexual enjoyment has many enemies, and there are many issues that continuously try to rob sexuality of its goodness. It's important to always remember that sexual happiness is no less valuable than anything else in our lives. Sexual happiness is not something to be neglected or ignored, but rather to be celebrated as one of the best things in life. Both members of a male-female relationship must find ways to keep the lust celebration going, no matter what.

The purpose of this book is to provide helpful ideas for rising above adversity and hanging on to the precious rewards of sexuality. Setting aside some time exclusively for sex for the sake of relationship and love is the idea. Every man and woman in relationship should occasionally set aside some time to immerse in sexual enjoyment—a special time, once or twice a year, to refurbish, reinvent, and rejuvenate the male-female relationships in the ambience of love. We need to forget the real world and devote time solely to the festive union of masculinity and femininity in a personal, secretive space. Couples should occasionally set aside time to take a wild ride to the depths of physical intimacy in search of new dimensions to their relationship, and to reflect on the goodness of a friendship in each other's arms amid the fragrance of love.

The idea presented here is a brief vacation—three to five days—for married couples, boyfriends and girlfriends, or special male-female friends. The purpose is to renew and rejuvenate the sex lives of women and men who are in committed companionship. We can call this an "Erocation" since it's an erotic vacation, or we can simply call it a" Hot Break". A Hot Break is when couples take a break from their regular day-to-day lives and go to a cozy, secluded place for a few days exclusively to enjoy sex with the intention of revitalizing their relationship. In a Hot Break, the focus is on physical intimacy and using sex to make couples more aware of how much they love each other.

It's true that most couples routinely take vacations, and that while on vacation, couples often get the opportunity to have sex, which might do some good in their relationship. The difference is that in most vacations, sexual enjoyment is just one among several possible activities. A typical vacation often includes children, other family members, relatives, and friends, and most vacation activities take place outside the hotel room or rental cottage.

But a Hot Break doesn't include children or anybody other than the man and woman themselves. Hot Breaks are intended solely to reinvigorate a couple's relationship. And the main event of the Hot Break happens inside the room; all other activities are secondary or can even be excluded if necessary. To the outside world, a Hot Break will look just like an ordinary vacation. Only the couple themselves knows they are on a Hot Break, as they discreetly enjoy their relationship in a special way.

The Hot Break will be presented step by step in the next few chapters. Follow the plan, but also allow yourselves the flexibility of making small changes to suit your unique circumstances and goals.

Eleven

The First Step to a Hot Break

There is one crucial step before entering into the details about what exactly should happen on a Hot Break. First, a sincere commitment and decision must be made. To achieve the goal, both members of the couple must demonstrate stern determination, total willingness, and an unshakable patience to go through all the steps to the very end. Only then should you undertake a Hot Break.

This step is critically important, because sexual enjoyment is often subconsciously considered to be of secondary importance. This is true of couples who have several children and are struggling financially to make ends meet, and that's understandable because survival must come first. However, we need to remember that there isn't much good in just being alive. We can spend our lives pretending that everything is great, even when we actually feel uncomfortable, unsatisfied, and unhappy, but our personal unhappiness often disrupts the quality of our external lives in ways that we don't realize. In a relationship, maintaining our personal happiness, physical intimacy, and sexual enjoyment is often more important than we simply think.

This is where Hot Breaks become relevant, because they are the best way for men and women in relationships to reclaim their personal happiness. A Hot Break is not just an opportunity for physical sexual enjoyment. The objective of a Hot Break is to tighten, rejuvenate, and rediscover the depths of love in a relationship by engaging in passionate sexual intercourse.

Women and men have problems that inhibit them from being fully aware of the status of their personal, secretive, inner happiness. When women move into their forties, the above mentioned inhibition grows rapidly for many of them if they're not really cautious. The reasons for this could be external, psychological, or even related to changes in their body chemistry. Whatever the reasons, women and men must be consciously determined to fight for their inner happiness before their lives become truly unhappy.

Many men fall into the trap of thinking that they shouldn't be concerned with matters of intimacy, whether romantic or psychological. Some men even think that engaging in such sentimentalities can weaken their masculinity, and this is a hard belief for some men to shake off. But it is possible if they can attain a real understanding of the facts and learn about the virtues of truly intimate relationships. The simple truth is that all men secretly crave soft love and appreciation. Men need to strip off their web of false beliefs and look at their intimate relationships with a fresh perspective, and going on a Hot Break is an ideal way to do that.

The decision to take a Hot Break must be mutual, resulting from a man and woman's mutual attraction and love for each other. The importance of a sincere, thoughtful decision to take action toward solving any serious problem is fully applicable with regard to the personal inner happiness of men and women in relationships.

For men and women who realize the importance of inner happiness in relationships, Hot Breaks will become meaningfully relevant. They will stubbornly decide to reignite their personal secret happiness, and Hot Breaks are the best way for men and women in committed relationships to do that. Adults of any age in a relationship must set aside some exclusive time once in a while to add fuel to the fire of their precious, personal, secret happiness. Celebrating wild sex soaked with love is the best way to achieve that goal, and a Hot Break is the perfect way to do it.

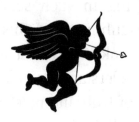

Twelve

Preparing for a Hot Break

Appropriate Time

The arrival of spring in the Northern Hemisphere, and six months later in the Southern Hemisphere, is like life getting a new beginning again and again. In the cool breeze of spring, fresh green leaves sprout and quickly grow on tree branches and bushes, and vast numbers of flowers begin to bloom in every color. All of these vibrant colors, along with the background music of chirping birds, are like a ceremony to welcome the summer. In the summer, the sun is bright and warm, the days are longer, it's easier to get around, and we can dress lightly—all of which makes it obvious that spring and summer are the best times of the year for a Hot Break.

But nothing stops anyone from taking a Hot Break during the winter either. In those cloudy gray days, especially when it's snowing, spending a Hot Break in a cozy and warm bedroom would be a special experience—secluded, romantic, and sensually mystic. If you feel like taking a Hot Break during the winter, go for it.

For those who live in tropical climates, any time of the year is good for a Hot Break. However, the rainy season might provide an extra special ambience of secluded, romantic coziness to a Hot Break in a carefully chosen location. The point is that although spring and summer are the best times to take Hot Breaks, if winter or the rainy season is the only time available, don't let that stop you.

Budget

Couples who have enough money for annual vacations don't have to worry about working out a meticulous budget to take a Hot Break; they just need the total plan. Since Hot Breaks are great for any adult who's in a relationship, most any couple can take a Hot Break once in a while if they really want to.

To hold down expenses, start by picking a location that's not too far from home, preferably a place easily reached by car or bus service. Don't stay at a luxury hotel or resort, because all of that luxury won't necessarily add much to a truly romantic Hot Break. In fact, too much luxury can become a distraction. Nevertheless, for people with plenty of money, there's nothing wrong with taking a Hot Break in a luxurious place if you're careful not to miss the actual purpose of being there.

If there's not much flexibility in your budget, an average motel at a peaceful location in a beautiful tourist town will be more than enough. Just don't try to save money by picking a small, deserted motel on the outskirts of town, because that could suck all the goodness right out of a Hot Break.

In planning your Hot Break, budget enough money so that you can enjoy nourishing, delicious food. If you'll have to be careful about every swipe of your credit card, leave the high-end lodgings and go for a midpriced option. Do some research to find a few good moderately priced restaurants in town, and that effort will probably lead to an exquisite dining experience at a surprisingly reasonable price.

Bed-and-breakfasts, hostels, and dormitories are not good for Hot Breaks. A couple's own house is not the best location for a Hot Break, but it can be a good second choice if your normal living space is available and free from any kind of intrusion. Most other aspects of a typical vacation will have little effect on your Hot Break budget.

Location

When searching for a Hot Break destination, there's no need to look for a place that offers outdoor activities. Your goal should be a peaceful, safe city or tourist town with a vibrant ambience, pleasant weather, and relatively good hotels and motels. A visually stunning small city or tourist location will enhance the mood of Hot Break.

Since your intention on a Hot Break is not sightseeing or attending a particular event, a location that's not too far from home and easy to reach is preferable, especially for those who are on a limited budget. If a couple is especially fond of a particular location, going to that place for Hot Break would be a good experience for them. If you live in a tropical area, try to go somewhere at a higher elevation with moderately cooler temperatures, such as a tourist hill station town.

Going on a tiresome two- or three-day trip to reach your Hot Break destination is not a smart idea. As you plan for your trip, always keep in mind the true purpose of your Hot Break.

A Hot Break Mystery

Imagine your few days of Hot Break as a mystical, erotic adventure, like a special hidden ritual involving a man and a woman in committed companionship. Experiencing the Hot Break as a secret vacation will make it even more enjoyable. This secretive approach will help you protect the goodness of Hot Break and avoid unnecessary embarrassments that could spoil this exceptional experience.

Couples will need to give their children, other family members, and friends an explanation for why they're going to be away from home for four or five days. If you're able to provide them with a factually true reason for being away, that's ideal. But the odds of that happening are extremely small, so your next-best option is to make up a believable story—with the one stipulation that nobody can possibly be hurt by it.

The ethics of telling a lie to achieve a good thing, such as the positive results of a Hot Break, are complicated. Since Hot Break is all about wild sex, which can happen only in private, it would be difficult to keep it secret any other way than making up a story. Nevertheless, fabricating a story for Hot Break can be tricky, so partners should discuss every detail of their story, accounting for anything that could go wrong, before finalizing and sharing it.

There are a few crucial things to remember in making up a story. Don't use relatives or friends known to your family in your story, since you can't ask them to cover for you. Also don't make up a story connected to your workplace or professional colleagues, because you can get caught in surprising ways.

Probably the best way to create a story is to build it around some kind of business project, for either you or your partner, that requires traveling to an actual place and meeting with some fictional people. (I'll resist providing more detailed suggestions to avoid the possibility of someone who knows you reading this book and stumbling across "your" story.) Drawing on your intelligence, common sense, and patience, create a story to fit your unique situation, and let the miracle happen in secrecy.

Fit Body

Hot Break will be a bit exhausting, because the main activity of Hot Break is having lots of physically demanding sex—not just the usual lazy intercourse. This doesn't mean that couples taking a Hot Break have to be in superb physical shape, like marathon runners or boxers. But a typically fit body capable of taking on some extra strain is a basic requirement for an enjoyable and rewarding Hot Break, so couples should make sure that they're in reasonably good shape. This generally won't be a concern for couples below the age of forty-five, but there could be an exceptional case when extra precautions regarding physical stress are necessary.

The point here is that all adults, particularly those above the age of forty-five, who plan to go on a Hot Break should make sure that they're in adequate shape to manage the physical strain of elaborate sexual intercourse sessions. Anyone who has a history of a problem such as heart disease, high blood pressure, diabetes, or muscle issues should confirm their body fitness by a qualified physician before going on a Hot Break.

One of the most important parts of the body for male-female relationships is the mouth, because kisses are the initial—and one of the most crucial—means of intimate physical connection. Partners' mouths must be clean and fresh, so that kisses can be passionately exchanged without any interruption or hesitation. To engage in a French kiss, oral hygiene and a pleasant mouth are absolutely necessary. If for some reason you haven't been to the dentist for your annual checkup and cleaning, that would be a good thing to do before packing up for a Hot Break. Gargling with mouthwash after brushing is the simplest way to keep the mouth healthy and fresh, and it's a good idea to take a bottle of mouthwash on your Hot Break.

Another important matter for men to check on while preparing for Hot Break is their penile erection potential. A fully erect penis is the basic tool that enables a man to achieve the most extreme level of physical intimacy with a woman. Penile erection capacity is crucial during a Hot Break because during the main activity, the penis has to remain erect for a longer period of time than during normal sexual intercourse. Men who are confident that their penile erection strength is normal don't need to worry about this, but those who have doubts should talk with a qualified physician. There's nothing wrong with depending on medications such as Viagra, Cialis, or Levitra for temporary help with penile erectile dysfunction, but you should do so only on the advice of your doctor.

Women must take into consideration the health of their vagina. Since it is the vagina that makes a woman capable of attaining the zenith of physical intimacy with a man, a healthy vagina is crucial in a physical relationship between a man and woman. One problem that can affect the vagina is dryness caused by insufficient natural lubrication, which can hinder the smooth entry of an erect penis and make sexual intercourse uncomfortable. Vaginal dryness typically develops during menopause because of a decrease in estrogen, although younger women occasionally experience vaginal dryness for other reasons.

Another serious problem that sometimes affects the vagina is pain (dyspareunia or vulvodynia) caused by some kind of infection. Vaginal pain can turn penile penetration during sexual intercourse into a painful nightmare for women. Vaginal dryness and pain are medically treatable, and over-the-counter lubricant creams can usually provide a quick temporary fix. But if you experience either of these problems, you also should consult with a qualified physician.

Normal sexual enjoyment can also be hampered by impotency in men and frigidity in women, which often result from a combination of physical and psychological issues. Treatment of these two problems, which should be done under the guidance of qualified physicians and psychotherapists, can be lengthy and complicated. Even though has to wait little longer and it is stressful it is worth to take that strain for a Hot Break.

A healthy, physically fit body will facilitate better lovemaking, and better lovemaking will make you more fit, and love will flourish in your fit body.

Groom the Body

To make the most of a Hot Break, the bodies of each partner must be well groomed and pleasing, which means taking care of a few things in advance. These might seem like negligible matters, but even a small issue can unexpectedly disrupt the flow of a Hot Break.

First, it's important that fingernails and toenails are short and that the edges of the nails are polished, because each partner will be using their fingers to play with soft and delicate parts of the other person's body. Men cannot take a lazy approach to this important matter, and women who grow longer nails for beauty reasons should find a convenient, comfortable way to manage this detail.

Another important aspect of grooming the body for Hot Break involves body hair—mainly pubic hair, armpit hair, mustaches, and beards. Simply removing hair from the armpits and pubic area is the best option, but having some hair won't be a problem. Men who wear a mustache and/or beard should take into consideration the comfort of their partners.

Contraception

Sometimes the primary purpose of sexual activity is to get pregnant, but that's not the goal of a Hot Break. The reason for going on a Hot Break is to strengthen the bond between a woman and a man and renew their love for each other by using or—perhaps more accurately—exploiting the extremely good feelings associated with sexual intercourse. Men and women on a Hot Break shouldn't have to worry about ending up with an unwanted pregnancy.

Fortunately several effective and safe means of contraception are now available. If used properly, condoms are the simplest and most effective way to avoid pregnancy. For women, contraceptive pills and IUDs (intrauterine devices inserted into the uterus) are good options, although they should be used only with the direction and help of a qualified physician. Obviously those who have taken advantage of a permanent sterilization method, such as a vasectomy or tubal ligation, don't need to worry about getting pregnant.

Adding a few packets of condoms to your baggage isn't a big deal. Just don't allow anxiety about getting pregnant to spoil the goodness of your Hot Break. On the other hand, for couples who want to conceive a child, the possibility of becoming pregnant can add an extra meaning to a Hot Break's celebration of sexuality.

Mood Music

Somehow music seems to be in the air when a woman and a man come together in romantic union. Good music can add an enjoyable ambience to a Hot Break, as anyone who has experienced romance knows. When you're preparing for a Hot Break, consider taking some music along to enhance this time of special intimacy with your partner. Most hotel and motel rooms won't have what you need, but you can take with you some CDs and a player, or just plan to use music available on the Internet. Nowadays most hotels and motels provide Internet access, although you might want to check before making reservations. YouTube makes it convenient to listen to two or three hours of romantic music, and all you need is a laptop and a small speaker.

Music can mysteriously enhance the romance of a sexual encounter between a man and a woman, but it's definitely not a requirement. The good things that happen on a Hot Break can take place just as well amid peaceful silence and sensuous murmurings. Some couples prefer to enjoy their own private erotic fantasies, wild and raw, and that's perfectly fine as long as it's a mutual agreement. Just don't miss out on the magic of music during a Hot Break because you weren't prepared.

Packing

Now it's time to pack for your Hot Break. Take as little luggage as possible, packing only the normal essentials for a short vacation. You won't need many clothes on a Hot Break, compared with a typical vacation. So pack just enough to meet your requirements, and keep your selections simple, light, cheerful, and suitable to the geography and climate of your Hot Break destination.

Don't forget to pack a few extra sheets, a small digital clock, any prescriptions that you regularly take, condoms, lubricants, and penile erection medication if needed. It's also a good idea to take a "Do Not Disturb" sign to hang on the outside door knob of your room, just in case you can't find one at the time of your Hot Break's main event.

Final Note

In all of your preparations for Hot Break, the most important thing is to have a healthy body. Hot Break won't be overly exhausting, but it will be longer and a bit more tiring than a normal intercourse session. As the author of this book, obviously I have no way of knowing about your physical health. Anyone who participates in a Hot Break, inspired by or using any of the ideas or illustrations presented in this book, must do so at their own risk and full responsibility.

Now your preparations are complete, everything is ready, and the time has come to head for your chosen location and begin the celebration of your very first Hot Break.

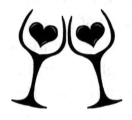

Thirteen

The First Day of a Hot Break

The first day of Hot Break starts with reaching the selected location: a beautiful tourist town or small city, probably facing a lake or sea and with a backdrop of amazing mountains that makes the place even more stunning and romantic. Ideally it will be a bright and sunny day, warm and breezy, an amorously perfect day for that place. Because the main ritual of Hot Break will take place inside, it does not matter whether it is rainy or shining outside. But if the days are bright and comfortable, and nights are pleasant, the overall experience of Hot Break will be more special.

The couple reaches their chosen Hot Break destination in their own vehicle, in a cab from the airport, or by bus or train. They arrive at the hotel or resort and check into their room, which is prepared and waiting for them. The couple enters their room with their luggage, the attendant leaves, the door is closed, and two pleasant sighs of relief mark the real beginning of Hot Break.

This first day of Hot Break is for total relaxing to let loose the mind and body, which have been strained for a while by the irritating monotony of day-to-day life and work. This is a day for the couple to settle into or enter into a time of whole Hot Break days on their own.

After arranging their belongings, they can order a simple drink such as tea, coffee, or something else, and if they are hungry, they can have a light snack as well. After enjoying that drink and bite, they can relax and rest for a short while lying on the bed. At this time the couple can exchange simple kisses and hug, but do not allow yourself to fall into the trap of being tempted to have sexual intercourse. No, absolutely not! You should keep all the extreme physical interactions for the main day of Hot Break, which is the next day. The first day of the Hot Break is only for relaxing and for knowing your Hot Break city or town, and to anticipate romance with a positive anxiety for the next day, the most important day of Hot Break.

After this short rest both partners freshen up, dress comfortably, and get out of the room to the streets. They walk around with people and move with the movements of the place, through the brightness of the day. When night falls, they mingle with the lights, and take in, inhale, and absorb the spirit of the place. Give yourselves to the vibe of that city or town. Let all the accumulated psychological toxins from worries, anxieties, and the stress of everyday living dissolve. Allow yourself to fully enjoy the freedom of this exclusive time with your closest special friend. With full willingness, give away your body and mind totally, falling into and dipping down into the brightness, movements, noises, colors, smells, and lights of this chosen place to enjoy with your beloved partner in this special secluded time.

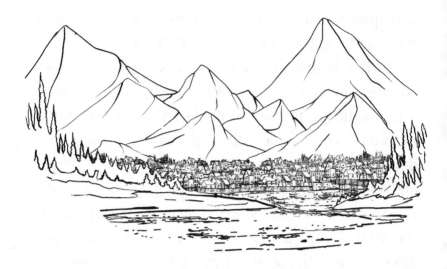

When you and your partner hold hands, smile, cuddle, and exchange kisses, only you two know what is going on and what you are really here for. Be in and enjoy the thrill of that secret and do not let loose the anxious anticipation about what is going to happen tomorrow.

The purpose of the first day of Hot Break is to dissolve all the stains and to melt away the rigidly wound-up layers of dark web caused by years of worries and anxieties about responsibilities and concerns about material security. Leave all the regrets about the past and all the worries and anxieties about the present and future behind where you live and work at least for these few days of Hot Break. Allow yourself to be in a carefree state with your partner to gain the whole goodness that can evolve out of this special time for an astonishing present and a better future.

Most men by nature are good at leaving the seriousness of real life aside and quickly getting into a carefree state of being. Most men have the ability to forget the things they have to worry about and to transition into party mode with ease. But females are naturally a bit incapable of ignoring the strains of the mind. This could be because they are more anxious about survival and curious about the future and security. This characteristic of femininity could be a basic requirement for life to go forward, taking care of things in proper balance to counter the bit of slackness men often have. But women must learn to disregard the serious things that cause anxiety and stress at least once in a while to escape that continuous invisible discomfort before it reaches a breaking point.

At this time of Hot Break, the woman must get into a carefree action mode so she does not miss any of the good things of Hot Break. The magic of Hot Break is going to do wonders.

After doing a joy wander around the town, the couple may get hungry. It is time to enjoy a nice restaurant. If possible, choose a restaurant exclusive to that particular city or town and have an elaborate lunch or dinner, depending on the time you two arrived, ignoring the hesitations of health consciousness. Eat the food slowly, consciously enjoying the taste. At this time of Hot Break, you can go a bit easy on the food budget. After finishing that nice meal, walk around through the streets where you didn't walk before. Then go to a green, flowery park and spend some time there or go to another special attraction of that place. At the end of the day, go to a place from which, ideally, you can enjoy a beautifully touching sunset in the nearness of your partner.

After the sun goes down and night falls, walk among the lights and shadows in a variety of hues, go to a nice restaurant again, and have a delightful dinner. Enjoy it at a relaxed, slow pace, relishing it thoughtfully with no hurry at all. Remember, consciously enjoying food passionately is an especially important part of the Hot Break celebration. Whenever you're finished with dinner, walk or take a cab back to your room.

Back in your room, soaked in the ambience of that town or city. Time has come for a good night's sleep to make ready your minds and bodies for the next day, the most important day of Hot Break.

Before comfortably settling into your cozy bed, there is a thing to deal with about the control of body and mind for the most crucial day of Hot Break. Orgasms or ejaculation will not be the priority tomorrow. Of course, there will be orgasms, but those are not going to be hurried. If that should be the situation, both partners must have lot of tolerance to keep their body and mind under good control, especially men. If the man has not ejaculated for a few days, keeping physical control to hold orgasm will be a hard task. The accumulation of semen will induce a natural pressure to let it out by orgasm.

If the male partner has not ejaculated for a few days and has a feeling of lustful pressure, the woman can give a simple hand job to her man to release the extra collected semen. That will make it easier for him to control his body with less strain of mind the next day.

Even though women do not accumulate body fluid like men that has to be gotten rid of to avoid sexual pressure, they also have a buildup of sexual pressure because of sex hormones. And if the woman has an untimely orgasm in the middle of Hot Break's important day, it will not be a disruption, because women possess the ability to enjoy multiple orgasms. But if giving a hand job makes the woman horny, the man can stimulate his woman's vagina and clitoris and by sucking her breasts can help her achieve a simple orgasm. There is nothing is wrong with it, but they absolutely should not have full sexual intercourse.

Both partners naturally will be perfectly tired now and can fall asleep. After simple kisses and cuddle and lights off, the couple can slide inside the sheets to sleep and sweet dreams.

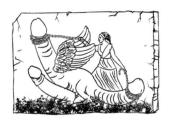

Chapter

Fourteen

The Most Important Day of a Hot Break

This is the day! Yesterday you left the monotony and stress of everyday life behind you, and last night your simple orgasms gifted you both with a sweet night's sleep. Now it's the morning of your most important day of Hot Break, so accept it with your whole heart. It makes no difference whether today is bright or overcast, sunny or rainy, because everything important is going to happen inside the four walls of your room. There's no need to wake up

97

early—but don't sleep too late, because you have many good things to do today.

While you're still in the bed, order something to drink—perhaps tea or coffee. Then get out of bed and enjoy your warm drink with great expectations for the day. Sit and relax for a few minutes, and then take turns performing your morning matters in the bathroom. Especially on this day, taking care of morning bathroom matters separately, one of you at a time, is strongly preferred. You want to save the intimate moments of togetherness for later in the day, to make this day special and exciting.

Being fresh and clean today is important. Take your clothes into the bathroom with you, and after taking a warm shower, get dressed simply and pleasantly. Then come out of the bathroom fully dressed. When choosing your clothes for today, avoid anything rough or thick with large buttons, or clothes with big knots or sharp pins. Even though only the two of you are in the room, keeping a fully clothed separation early in the day will increase your enjoyable anxiety about what is going to happen later. Now that you're clean and fresh, dressed in simple clothing, order whatever each of you wants for breakfast and enjoy your meal together. After your nice breakfast, just relax and chat for awhile.

Especially today, neither of you should try to impose anything on the other. Instead, you should enthusiastically try to make your partner happy. Keep in mind, with sincerity and total willingness, the magic verse for today is: "Making you happy makes me happy." Each of you should cherish seeing the other one happy, without worrying about your own happiness. When "Making you happy makes me happy" is working in both directions, you will be automatically bestowed with happiness. Let the effect of this magic verse surround you as you go through the day.

What Is It About Today?

This is the most important day of Hot Break because of what's going to take place later—a detailed and elaborate session of extreme physical intimacy and sexual intercourse between a woman and a man passionately committed to each other. This is going to be an indoor sexual roller coaster, a wild sex ride. As your bodies become fused in passion, an abundance of lovemaking will immerse you in an aura of love that will quench your yearning for sexual happiness.

In a situation like this, your anticipation of sexual happiness might significantly raise your expectations. That's normal, because the feeling of sexual enjoyment is naturally an extremely intense experience. Just be careful not to lose patience, because this wild sex ride will take at least two to three hours. Both of you must give yourselves to each other during this time with total willingness, relax, let go of your body, and enter with your whole personality into this special time.

It's important to jointly agree on an appropriate time of day that is comfortable for both of you. The best time to begin this special ritual of lovemaking is in the morning between nine and ten o'clock, and it will last until noon or one o'clock in the afternoon. After the making-love celebration, you can have a cozy nap, after the nap can go out to have a fabulous lunch. The second-best option is to start the ritual of making love in the afternoon between two and three o'clock, and it will last up to five or six o'clock in the evening. After that passionate lovemaking ritual and a short rest, you can go out for a multi course dinner and enjoy the rest of the evening. It's not a good idea to begin your lovemaking ritual later than six o'clock in the evening, because you'll be more tired than earlier in the day.

If you together decide to perform the passion ritual of lovemaking in the morning, you can begin your preparations shortly after breakfast. If you pick the afternoon, begin your preparations after a simple, light lunch.

As you begin preparing for the erotic ceremony, if you have children, first contact them and make sure that they're fine, because your peace of mind is important. Then arrange with the front desk not to connect any calls to your room for at least four hours, and give them a plausible reason for this request. Unless you have children, turn off your cell phones. Let all the powers of the universe protect you from any disturbances during this wonderful time of your lives.

Hang the "Please Do Not Disturb" card on your doorknob and lock the door. Turn on your chosen music and close the windows and curtains. Adjust the lighting to achieve an appropriate mood, according to the preferences of both partners. You might want to turn on the bathroom light and keep that door open a bit, and some daylight will also filter through the drapes or curtains.

The room temperature should be between twenty-three and twenty-five degrees centigrade, or whatever you both find comfortable. A lukewarm surrounding would be suitable for this auspicious occasion. Then spread the sheets you brought on the bed, and place your lubricants, condoms, and tissues within easy reach for when you need them.

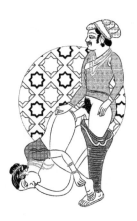

Fifteen

The First Hug

Finally the time has come and the mood has been set by appropriate lighting and temperature. Beautiful music slowly fills the room, piercing the secret world of your two hearts. Good music can magically transform any surroundings into a cozy imaginary place, and this soothing music will shift you into that place filled with warm emotions.

As you stand facing each other, gently join hands and slowly draw each other closer. It's impossible to live every moment of our lives like this, but when you have this opportunity, don't take it for granted. As the romantic music starts to work its magic on you, pull closer and wrap your arms firmly around each other. Look into each other's eyes with pure fascination and a total lack of reasoning. This will turn into a strong and passionate hug—the first hug of the amazing ceremony of lovemaking on the most crucial day of Hot Break.

Lovingly kiss each other now—a long kiss enjoyed with total acceptance. After a minute or so, slowly pull out of the kiss, close your eyes, and hug each other closely. Stay glued firmly together, not letting go or opening your eyes. As you kiss and hug, be careful not to hurt each other; the man should be especially careful toward the woman.

Enjoy the exquisite presence and fullness of being held in your beloved one's arms. This is the time to let good memories bubble up about this person to whom you are closer than anyone else in the whole world. Let all those beautiful memories roll around in every nook and cranny of your mind. Do not entertain even one negative thought about the person inside your arms during this amazing time of love. Don't allow anything to spoil this moment as you delight in the warmth of the flesh that fills your arms, where the soul of your beloved one dwells. Relish its fullness, take it all in, and let this priceless good feeling pour into your soul. Enjoy this goodness thoughtfully, clearly, and consciously, as much and as long as you want.

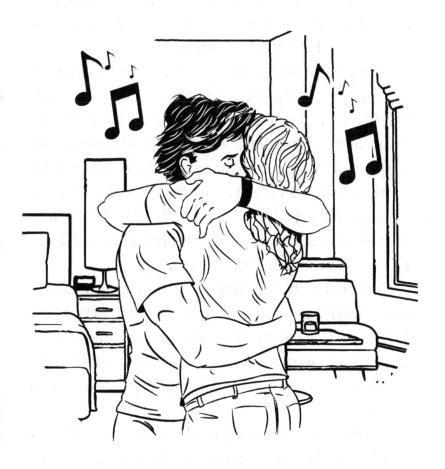

There are only two thin layers of clothing between you. Let it be that way for now—nothing erotic or sensual. That first hug allowed you to enjoy the wholesomeness of your most beloved one inside your arms physically and as a person. Enjoy passionate kisses now and then, but be careful not to slip into an urgent need for sexual gratification.

The goal of this unusual ceremony of lovemaking is not just to have an orgasm or relieve sexual tension by ejaculating, but to enjoy your relationship with your beloved one in emotional and physical wholeness. The purpose of this particular segment is to emotionally relish the physical presence of your most beloved one inside your tightly wrapped arms. There will be waves of intense orgasms later, but for now, move patiently through this amazing experience.

Continuing that first hug, move your arms smoothly and affectionately all over your beloved one's body. Run your fingers through their hair and move your arms slowly across their shoulders, arms, back, sides, and buttocks, feeling and enjoying it clearly and consciously.

As romantic music flows all around you both, let go of the tightness of your mind and body and freely immerse yourself in this romantic, mystical ambience. Continue this way for at least fifteen minutes, totally immersed and involved. Enjoy with desire your beloved one's presence, holding one another tightly, close inside each other's arms for as long as you want. Your heart will not be easily satisfied; it will yearn for more and more.

Just be there for awhile, holding tightly to your beloved one. Take all of that feeling deep into your soul for fifteen, twenty, even twenty-five minutes. Then slowly move to the second segment of this fascinating ceremony of lovemaking.

Sixteen

The Second, "Stark" Hug

The two of you are now in a mystical but real world. This is not just a fantasy—it's really happening. Nobody in the outside world will ever know what is truly going on here in your private world.

As you stand there, your hearts are getting soft from the sweetly piercing music that whirls all around. Now it's time for each of you to unbutton or unzip the top half of the other's clothing, sliding it down and smoothly exposing shoulders and then chests and breasts. Gently hug each other again, letting the happiness of that hug seep into your hearts. Stay in that sweet hug for at least five minutes. Then slowly pull back a bit, remove the rest of your partner's clothing, and toss it somewhere out of the way.

Now you are standing stark naked, with nothing to hide, in front of your closest human being in this world. The totally naked you is the real you. Generally people are able to be their true selves, physically or emotionally, only in private. Sometimes they can be themselves in front of a few other people, but often only with one person. That's what is happening now. In this situation, you have an amazing opportunity to be yourself and to experience and relish the closest person in your life almost completely as themselves.

The only things that can spoil this auspicious occasion of lovemaking are inhibitions, shyness, and vulnerability anxiety. Both of you must shed all physical and psychological inhibitions, shyness, and vulnerability anxiety in front of this person whom you completely trust by totally relaxing your body and mind. This can work the other way around as well: When you totally relax your body and mind and expose yourself, you automatically become acceptable to the other person. When you let every trace of inhibition, shyness, and vulnerability anxiety melt away, you'll start to experience a wonderful freedom in being naked. Your nakedness will also generate an interesting feeling of truthfulness and a thrill that you don't have any secrets from the person closest to you.

After removing your clothes, don't remain separated for more than a minute or two. Holding hands, pull toward each other again into the second, "stark" hug. Wrap your arms tightly around one another as though trying to merge into each other, and devour the intense good feeling of togetherness. Still standing, move slowly to the music while kissing and sliding your hands all over your beloved one.

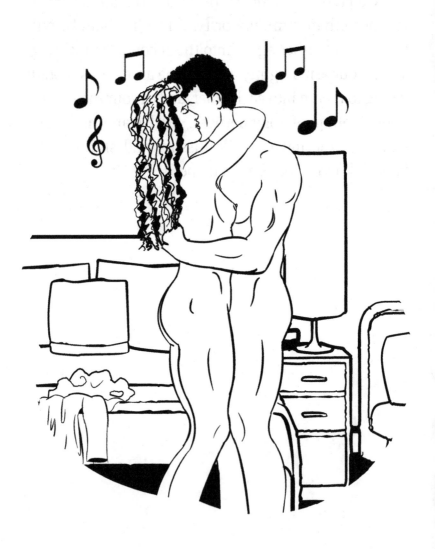

The stark hug is different from the first hug. In a stark hug, nothing separates you. Your body and skin are in direct contact with your most intimate one's body and skin. It feels as though your skin is emitting its texture, smoothness, warmth, and presence through your partner's skin and into the body, and the same thing happens the other way around as well. Now your beloved one will be radiating all the characteristics and warmth of their skin and body through your skin and into your body. If you close your eyes and keenly concentrate on the feeling of this skin-to-skin interaction, it's truly an amazing experience.

Don't hurry through this embrace. Slowly and thoughtfully take in the whole presence of your partner's body through your skin. Continue moving one hand, slowly and smoothly, all over your beloved one's body—from hair to shoulders, arms, back, sides, buttocks, and thighs. Consciously enjoy the feeling absorbed through your fingers, while you hug them tightly with your other hand. Switch hands now and then, sometimes caressing your partner continuously, sometimes embracing them tightly with both hands. There are no rigid rules; just do whatever you both comfortably enjoy, including standing totally still in an intimate embrace.

In this segment of the amazing ceremony of lovemaking, things will become more sensuous. Now you will more explicitly feel your partner's breasts, nipples, chest, erect penis, pubic hair, vagina, or testicles.

But both of you must patiently remain in total control, because you aren't yet anywhere close to engaging in sexual intercourse. This segment, the "stark" hug, allows you to relish the whole presence of each other's body through the extreme intimacy of skin in a firm embrace.

Let this continue for awhile, sticking together firmly in direct skin-to-skin connection and enjoying the feeling. This skin-to-skin intimacy will create a heartwarming feeling in both bodies. Relish it passionately as you exchange kisses, and continue in the presence and warmth of your beloved one's body by running your hands slowly all around.

After ten to twelve minutes, walk slowly to a loveseat or couch, delighting in the nakedness of each other without any inhibition or shyness. Imagine that the music circling around is actually propelling you there. The man sits down first, his penis possibly erect by now. Paying not that much attention to her partner's penis, but very carefully the woman sits across his thighs and tightly embraces him in an intimate hug. Continue in this extremely impassioned embrace until your hearts feel full.

When your breasts or penis rub against skin, you might become sexually aroused, but remember that this most important day of Hot Break is not just about two orgasms. Ignore the touching of nipples and penis for now, and concentrate fully on the skin-to-skin connection and warmth of this "stark" hug." Take it all into your hearts joyously.

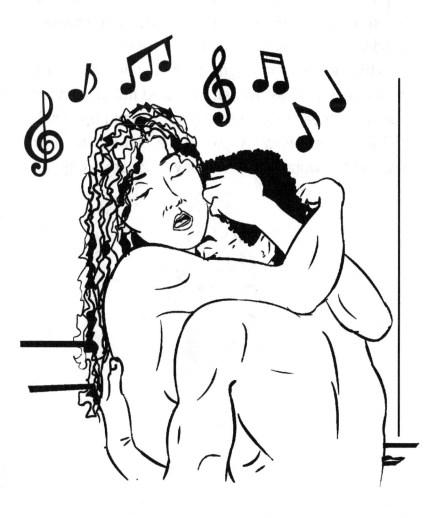

While glued together in this embrace, let your bodies slide against each other and your hands caress each other to heighten the feeling. Take this special opportunity to let your love for your beloved one bloom in all the colors in your heart, as you silently ponder positive thoughts and secret apologies.

This "woman on thighs of man" variation of the "stark" hug can last for ten to fifteen minutes. When you're both eager to move forward, stand up slowly and let the music carry you to the bed for the third stage of the wonderful ceremony of lovemaking.

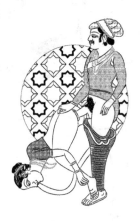

Chapter

Seventeen

Amorous Massage

Walk to the bed as though possessed by music, either the real music around you or the romantic music of your heart. Holding each other closely, crawl onto the bed, roll each other over, and exchange a deep kiss. Now it's time to let your emotions fire up and become more erotic. From here on, don't allow the sensuous momentum to drop.

As per the usual practice, ladies first. After the kiss, let the female partner turn over and lie face down on the bed. This third segment of the wonderful ceremony of lovemaking, the massage, will be somewhat physically demanding. So both partners should be mentally prepared, their hearts filled with love, and willing to endure some physical strain to make your beloved one happy.

As mentioned earlier, the most important magic verse for this Hot Break—and especially for this most important day—is "Making you happy makes me happy." The magic verse can be simply explained as "I am joyfully enjoying whatever I am doing, as long as what I'm doing makes you happy." Both partners should recite the first magic verse silently in their minds every now and then throughout this most important day of Hot Break, especially from here on. This first magic verse, "Making you happy makes me happy," should be very active in the minds of both partners, particularly during this segment on the amorous massage.

The amorous massage is specifically intended for waking up all the receptacles of the bodies of both partners, from head to toe, so that you can receive and fully enjoy all the goodness of the wonderful ceremony of lovemaking. Partners are going to give each other a loving, wholesome, total massage, and each partner should enter into the amorous massage with passion and a willingness to give.

Both of you are in the bed now, and the woman is lying face down with her eyes closed. The man straddles her, facing her head and placing his knees on either side of her body without resting the full weight of his body on her back. Softly hovering over her, begin to slowly massage her head, neither too firmly nor too feebly, with an eagerness to make her feel really good. Continue massaging all over your beloved partner's head in circular movements with all ten fingertips. After three to four minutes, slide your hands slowly down to her neck.

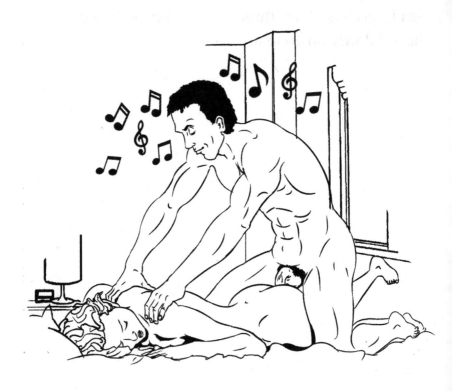

Start to gently massage your partner's neck, keeping your fingers together, in circular or zigzag movements. Many arteries, veins, nerves, and vital ducts pass through her neck, so be careful and gentle. Continue massaging in a slow rhythm and be happy that you are making your woman happy. You should enjoy her happiness. After pleasuring her neck for two or three minutes, slowly come down to her shoulders.

Now start massaging from the bottom of her neck toward her shoulders, moving both of your hands back and forth slowly and lovingly. Smoothly rub and roll in zigzag or circular movements, keeping your fingers together. Gently squeeze the flesh on both sides of her neck. Change your movements from time to time, but be careful not to hurt your partner and disrupt her enjoyment. This caution should be in the minds of both partners throughout this amorous massage and for the whole wonderful ceremony of lovemaking.

When the man lovingly labors to evoke joy in his partner's body by massaging her, the woman focuses her whole consciousness on the precious sensation of his hands, wholeheartedly relishing the good feelings that he is creating. The man continues to patiently massage the woman's neck and shoulders for two to three minutes, and then allows his hands to drift down to her upper arms.

The man continues massaging the woman's upper arms, from shoulder to elbow, smoothly squeezing and pressing. Please her by sliding both of your hands back and forth over one of her arms at a time. Slowly come down to her lower arms, and massage all the way down to her fingers. Then go back to her lower arms and then to her upper arms, all the way squeezing and pressing in a pleasing rhythm. Do this to both of her arms a few times, for three to four minutes.

As the man does this, the first magic verse, "I am joyfully enjoying whatever I am doing to make you happy," should be active in his mind. When you really enjoy the act of making your partner happy, you'll be amazed at what a good feeling it is.

After pleasuring the woman's arms for three to four minutes, the man can shift himself further back and drag both of his hands softly to her upper back. As you hover and move around over your partner's body, remember to maintain a connection to her skin. You can softly drag your testicles, penis tip, and buttocks across her body, like a secondary massage, while continuing to make her happy with your hands. The feel of your penis, testicles, and buttocks moving over her skin will be an interesting, intimate experience for her.

The man should now start massaging the woman's upper back slowly, moving both hands up and down in circular and zigzag movements. Use a combination of love squeezes and pressure, always being careful not to hurt her. Continue creating good feelings, massaging from her upper back to the middle of her back with passion and imagination. Do this a few times, and then let your fingers slide down toward the base of her breasts and massage softly with great care for some time. Then move your fingers back up to her mid and upper back, and move back and forth several times, massaging her breasts, sides, and back.

Meanwhile the woman should lie calmly, eyes closed, body fully relaxed, completely giving yourself to your partner and letting him make you happy. Take his gift into your heart and enjoy it, concentrating on the wonderful feeling of his hands massaging every part of your body.

As the man creates happiness in the woman's body, his mind must remain clearly focused on his palms and fingertips, relishing the feel of her skin and the wholeness of her flesh. As you massage her, don't forget to maintain the secondary pleasure of touching her with your penis, testicles, and buttocks. After massaging her upper back, mid back, sides, and breasts for three to four minutes, it's time to turn around.

The man now slowly and carefully shifts his legs to the opposite sides, hovering over the woman's body without lowering his full weight onto her body and being careful not to hurt her. Do this as quickly as possible, so as not to interrupt the woman's enjoyment. Now facing her legs, begin massaging her lower back in circular and zigzag movements with both hands, holding your fingers straight. Take a few minutes to patiently massage her lower back and both sides.

Now you've reached one of the most erotic, gorgeous parts of a woman's body, her buttocks. You're going to treat your partner's buttocks as though they're two beautiful balls of dough that need to be conditioned to perfection. If we were actually working with dough, we would refer to this process as *kneading*—but we'll just call it *doughing* instead.

The man should now slowly start doughing both of your partner's soft buttocks, lovingly rotating, pressing, and zigzagging across all sides, curves, and grooves. Your movements should be slow and long, because fast-paced agitation in sexually sensitive areas such as the buttocks, which are close to the vagina, may increase sexual tension in woman. An eager urgency to achieve orgasm would spoil your slow, patient enjoyment of the wonderful ceremony of lovemaking in its wholeness.

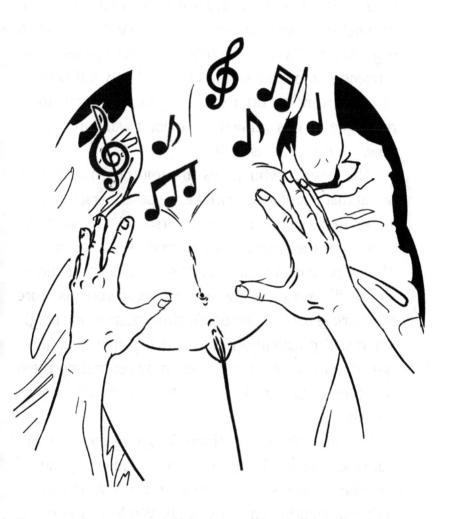

Now it's time for the second magic verse of the most important day of Hot Break. This verse has two versions: the person receiving an amorous massage says, "I don't want an orgasm now," and the person giving the amorous massage says, "We don't want an orgasm now." When the man reaches to pleasure an erogenous zone, the woman must silently tell herself, "I don't want an orgasm now." And the man must recite the giver's version, "We don't want an orgasm now," in his mind as well.

The person who gives an amorous massage is doing that out of love to make the other person happy, so it's more suitable for that person to use the "we" version of the second magic verse. But the receiver of an amorous massage needs more physical control, so the "I" version of the second magic verse is more appropriate for that person. Reciting this second magic verse will drastically reduce the urgency to achieve orgasm in both men and women by reminding them that they didn't go on a Hot Break just to have two orgasms.

The man should continue doughing the woman's buttocks with kisses and love squeezes, doing rotations, zigzags, and whatever other movements his wild imagination can dream up. While this is going on, the woman should continue to concentrate on whatever part of her body feels good at the moment, absorbing it all and consciously enjoying it. The man should focus on the good feeling experienced by his palms and fingers by the woman's soft, warm buttocks and continue doughing for two to three minutes

Next the man slowly and smoothly shifts to the back of the woman's thighs, pleasuring her by pressing, zigzagging, rolling, and squeezing back and forth from one leg to the other. Then move to her knees, her lower legs, and down to her heels, continuing to roll, zigzag, press, and squeeze with the sincere goal of evoking good feelings. After a minute or two, return to her knees and the backs of her thighs and make them happy again, and then repeat this cycle—thighs to knees to lower legs to heels—a few times with patience and willingness to make your woman happy. This pleasuring of the backs of the woman's legs can take about three minutes. The man then smoothly slides his hands back up to the woman's buttocks and does more doughing for a minute.

Then the man flips his partner over so that she's lying on her back, as the woman keeps her eyes closed. The woman is now lying in front of the man, stark naked, presenting her whole physical and psychological entity to be pleasured by him. The man again straddles the woman, facing her head with his knees on either side of her body, without putting his full weight on her. Since the front of a woman's body is softer and less muscular than her back, the man must now be more careful. He can continue, however, to maintain a sensual connection by touching her with his penis, testicles, and buttocks.

The man now bends forward and lovingly places one hand on each side of his partner's face. In doing so, he is openly accepting, with an open heart, the woman's personality and identity in its wholeness by adoring her face. This face adoration has meaning only if you're able to forgive and discard all complaints and grudges against your partner. Only good memories and thoughts of her can be allowed to flow in and fill your heart. If you can adore your partner's face with a clear, positive mind, you will experience a distinctive kind of joy—the joy of really loving someone. This adoration of your partner has nothing to do with her face's beauty, color, shape, or age. It's about who she really is, how she fascinates you, and why you appreciate that.

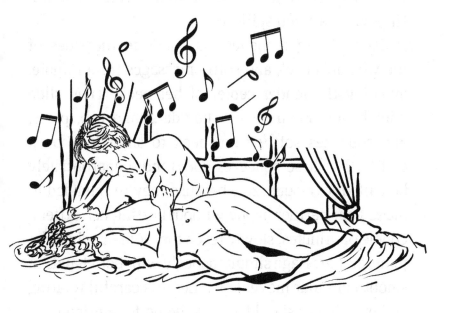

Gently holding his beloved partner's face in his hands, the man stoops down and kisses her forehead, eyes, nose, and cheeks, and finally her lips as well. This should not be a sensuous French Kiss—save that for later. Then using your fingertips, softly caress her face and ear lobes softly for a couple of minutes, continuing to adore her face and evoke pleasure in her. Enjoy your feeling of love for your partner and let it fill your heart and spill over.

Next the man moves his hands to the sides of the woman's neck and softly massages for a minute, avoiding the tender center of her neck. Then slide your hands down to her shoulders, and rub, press, and squeezes softly from neck to shoulders, back and forth. These squeezes could more appropriately be called love squeezes, because they're intended to make your partner happy without hurting her. After a couple of minutes, slowly reach the woman's shoulder joints and massage simultaneously with both hands in smooth circular movements. Let this careful rotating and pressing of shoulder joints go on for a minute.

Sliding your hands down to your partner's upper arms, massage them with rotations, presses, and love squeezes. Continue this process, moving to her elbows, lower arms, and then her fingertips. Then move back and forth several times between her shoulders and her fingertips, massaging both arms with rotations, presses, and love squeezes. When you reach her shoulders for the third or fourth time, stop and let your palms crawl slowly toward your partner's breasts.

Most men love women's breasts and consider them the most beautiful objects in the world. On the most important day of Hot Break, your partner's beautiful breasts will stimulate you to the next level of sexual enjoyment. Taking one of your beloved woman's breasts in both hands, adore it lovingly for a while, and then do the same with the other breast. Now, being especially careful, perform doughing on both breasts, smoothly and slowly moving back and forth from one to the other. Shower kisses all over your beloved woman's mammary balls, suck both of her nipples, and run your fingertips over her areola rings with passion but softly. Do doughing on both breasts with zigzags, rolls, shakes, and love squeezes, smoothly and with great care. Enjoy the fullness and softness of her breasts in your hands and the satisfaction of making your woman happy. Meanwhile, don't forget to maintain the connection between your partner's body and your penis, testicle sack, and buttocks.

The woman should not get distracted and miss any of the good feeling that your beloved man generates as he doughs your breasts. Take it all in and relish it with clear concentration and an inner gratitude for his love.

While doughing his partner's breasts, the man should be careful to maintain a slow rhythm and avoid creating in her a sexual urgency for orgasm.

Breasts are highly erogenous, so the best way for both of you to be in control is to use the two versions of the second magic verse. For the woman, "I don't want an orgasm now," and for the man, "We don't want an orgasm now."

From here on, a third magic verse is also used: "Slow and long." As both partners begin to deal with erogenous zones more intimately, avoiding urgency for sexual relief through orgasm is important to enjoy the wholeness of the wonderful ceremony of lovemaking. So whenever you reach an erogenous zone, remember to use the third magic verse, "Slow and long," and keep all massage movements slow and long.

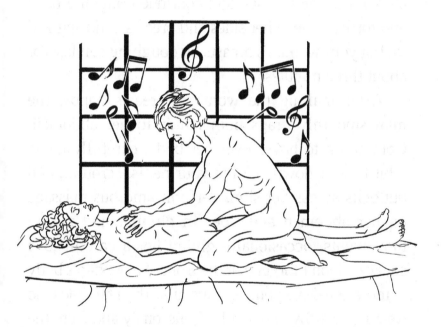

The man continues doughing both of the woman's breasts one after the other, or he can simultaneously place one palm on each breast and lovingly knead her two love balls to perfect condition. Don't neglect the sides of the body where her breast bases are. Carefully massage with both hands smoothly along the bases of both breasts, slowly rotating down to the bed and then back up to the breasts, and continue doughing back and forth between her sides and breasts. Adoring and loving your woman's breasts by doughing can last for about three minutes.

After making the woman's breasts happy, the man smoothly drags both hands to her abdomen. Continuing to hover over her body, carefully move a bit further down, sliding your penis, scrotum, and buttocks across her skin. Perform amorous massage on her abdomen and sides in circular and zigzag movements, occasionally giving her a careful love squeeze. Don't forget that the front of a woman's body is more sensitive and less muscular than her back, so treat it carefully and gently. Generously and from the bottom of your heart, continue pleasing your woman's belly and around both sides of her body with long and slow movements.

The man now moves to one side of the woman's body and assumes a comfortable, balanced position close to her naked body. Without a long pause, continue to perform amorous massage on her belly, lower belly, and groin area, being careful not to lose your balance and put your full weight on her. For a couple of minutes, create happiness in your beloved woman's belly. When you move close to her groin area, intentionally avoid the vagina for now. The vagina is the pinnacle of a woman's body with regard to lovemaking, so you must deal with your partner's vagina with great care and special delight.

After pleasing your woman's lower belly, slide your palms slowly to her legs. Please her thighs, one after the other, with love squeezes, presses, rolls, and zigzags. After a little while, shift to her knees, her lower legs, and finally her heels and toes. Just as you did on the backs of her legs, repeat this hip to toe pleasure glide two or three times. Meanwhile you can switch to either side of the woman's body so that you're comfortable, and patiently give your woman's legs a loving treat.

Now the time has come to take care of your partner's vagina. Men find women's vaginas to be very mysterious. They seem outwardly simple—just a fleshy, triangular bulge with a small slit in the middle, decorated by beautiful curly pubic hair and perched right where her sexy thighs meet. Internally, however, the vagina is a sophisticated organ. Even adolescent boys know that something mysterious hides between women's legs, but it's not until adulthood that they learn that a woman's vagina possesses an amazing ability to bestow on them an intensely wonderful feeling. But don't waste time trying to figure it out. Just hurry up and enjoy all the happiness your woman's vagina has to offer.

The man should now spread the woman's legs slightly apart and take a kneeling position between them. As your hands converge at your partner's ultimate pleasure center, her vagina, place your palms, without much pressure, on either side of the vaginal opening close to her labia majoras. Labia majoras are the most external parts on either side of the vaginal opening. Enjoy the view of your woman's vagina as though you've never before seen it. Slowly start to move your palms up and down. Holding your fingers together, rub and squeeze both labia majoras lovingly and smoothly with great care without agitating the clitoris.

Since the vagina is the most sensitive erogenous zone in a woman's body, all of your movements should be "slow and long." As mentioned earlier, you don't want to develop an urgent eagerness for orgasm in your partner. Here again it is time for both partners to use their respective versions of the second magic verse. The man should think, "We don't want an orgasm now," and the woman must tell herself, "I don't want an orgasm now."

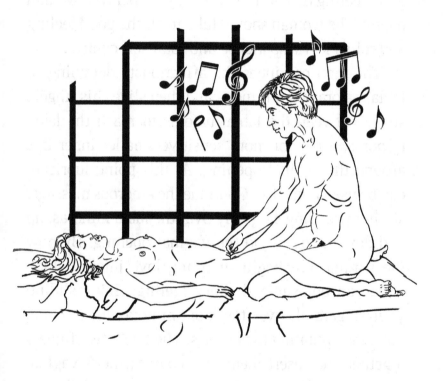

Continue performing amorous massage on her labia majoras with zigzags and love squeezes. Then let it slowly turn into full doughing, but use long, slow movements that extend now and then up to her hip joints and lower abdomen. The man should not miss the subtle romantic music ambience and enjoy the good feeling that you're making your beloved woman happy. The woman should take in all the good feeling and relish it with patience and total self control.

The man continues the affectionate doughing of labia majoras for a minute, and then slides his fingers softly between the labia majoras to reach the labia minoras, a pair of more sensitive smaller inner lips around the vaginal opening. At this point, lubricant can be used if needed. Continue the amorous massage, sliding your fingers gently over the labia minoras, up and down and around the vaginal opening. By now the vagina will begin secreting love juices, which create an enjoyable slippery feeling. Enjoy sliding your fingers all over the labia minoras for a while, but avoid agitating the clitoris. Then hold two fingers together and insert them into your partner's vagina, moving slowly in and out and rotating carefully and lovingly. During this vaginal doughing, shift your position from between the woman's legs to the left or right side of her hip.

Make the labia minoras and vaginal opening happy for a while, and then lovingly rotate your fingers in and out of the vaginal opening. After a little while, return to doughing the external vagina with zigzags and love squeezes, then again go in and make the labia minoras and vaginal duct happy, and so on. Go back and forth a few times, using slow movements and avoiding stimulating the clitoris much or hurting your beloved woman.

After the man has enjoyed this naughty sensuous game with his partner's vagina for several minutes, slowly drag both hands away and move upward, rubbing your fingers smoothly through the mons pubis, lower abdomen, upper abdomen, breasts, shoulders, and neck. Finally surround your beloved woman's face inside your palms and give her a love kiss with an overflowing heart, and then slowly lie down beside her.

The woman should take a few seconds to absorb that kiss. Then open your eyes and slowly roll onto your man's body, take his face in your hands, and give your beloved man a love kiss with passionate gratitude, enjoying the warmth of your partner's body and the passion in the air, surrounded by romantic music for a while. Then move down to the bed and lie beside your man.

The man now turns around and lies face down on the bed. It's his turn now to receive an amorous massage.

Eighteen

Amorous Massage: The Man's Turn

The time has come for the man to be immersed in the treat of an amorous massage, so after the gratitude kiss, he flips over and lies face down. In this situation, his penis might be partially or even fully erect, which could make it inconvenient for him to lie on his stomach. But beds are usually rather soft, so he should be able to overcome this problem.

Facing his head, the woman straddles the man's body. You can rest some of your weight on your partner's body, because generally men are physically stronger than women. Sit with your soft buttocks resting gently on his back, but make sure that you're not hurting him. Let the first magic verse, "Making you happy makes me happy," keep running through your head as you begin creating happiness in your beloved man's body. But also keep your senses keenly receptive to the wonderful feelings that are about to pass through your palms and fingers.

The man presents himself totally to his beloved partner and prepares to absorb all of the good feelings that she's about to create in his body. Concentrating your mind on the exact points of your body where your woman's palms and fingers are working.

The woman now begin the amorous massage with her partner's head, burying her fingers in his hair and evoke pleasure by pressing, rubbing softly, and rotating her fingers against his scalp. Meanwhile don't miss the opportunity to connect to your man's body with your soft buttocks, touches of your wet vagina, and brushing against your pubic hair. Leaving love stains with your wet vagina all over your man's body will surely be an exciting sensual experience for him, so maintain this connection throughout the amorous massage.

There is little difference between a woman's amorous massage of a man and a man's amorous massage of a woman. After pleasing your man's head for awhile, softly rub his neck and then move to his shoulders with presses, love squeezes, and zigzags. Evoke happiness in his shoulders, and then move to his shoulders and make them happy with loving rotations. Then please his arms with rolls and love squeezes, and massage one arm after the other, back and forth from shoulder joints to fingertips. Women can follow the detailed massage suggestions in the previous chapter, simply adopting any changes necessitated by the gender reversal.

After spending enough time on his arms, move to his upper back, mid back, and sides, using your imagination to create amorous massage movements that your man will thoroughly enjoy. After about three minutes, turn around to face his feet and continue the amorous massage on his lower back and eventually his sexy buttocks.

Here's the woman's first chance for doughing on her partner's body. Women have four erogenous points on their bodies for doughing: lips, breasts, vagina, and buttocks. But men have only three—lips, genitals, and buttocks—unless you also include male nipples. The woman can now delight her partner by lavishly doughing his buttocks with various massage movements while playfully enjoying herself as well. Happily perform doughing on your man's buttocks for two or three minutes. Then move close to one of his legs and massage the backs of his thighs with presses, zigzags, love squeezes, and rotations. Next massage his knees, lower leg muscles, and his heels, and move back and forth between his hips and heels several times.

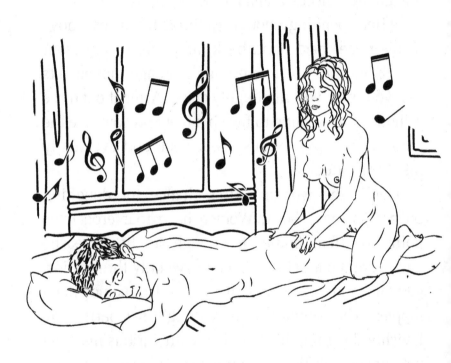

After pleasing the backs of your man's legs, slide your palms slowly back to his buttocks and resume doughing. Meanwhile your partner should be concentrating on the exact points from where the good feeling is coming and not miss a bit of it. Dough your man's buttocks for a little while longer and then move your hands away.

The man now flips over and lies on his back with his eyes closed. Without much of a pause, the woman takes a position above his lower chest and carefully re-establishes her connection to him with her soft buttocks and wet vaginal touches.

The amorous massage on the front of the man's body begins with face adoration, just as it did with the woman's body. When the woman adores the man's face, she accepts him with her whole heart, forgives his shortcomings, and keeps any complaints about him far away from their Hot Break site. She recognizes that he is just a human being incapable of being perfect every second of his life. Adoring the man's face is not about its appearance, but about accepting him for who he really is. Face adoration is truly a matter of love.

In a situation such as a Hot Break, a woman should just love her man. Don't waste time tallying his merits. Just enjoy the pleasure of giving your love to him whether he deserves it or not. Real love is not something that happens in back and forth negotiations. Real love is freely and selflessly giving your heart to someone, with a high probability that you'll get that love back many times over.

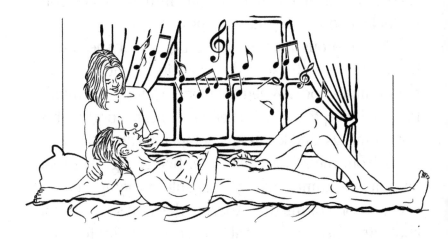

The woman now cradles the man's face in both of her hands, bends over, and spreads soft kisses—not yet deep and sensuous—all over his forehead, eyes, cheeks, nose, chin, and lips. After the kisses, rub his ear lobes softly between your fingers for a little while. Then slide your fingers up to his forehead, rub and zigzag tenderly, and smoothly and lovingly do the same all over his face for a couple of minutes.

Then pull your hands down to his shoulders and evoke pleasure there with a variety of massage movements. After spending a couple of minutes there, please his arms and then move back to his chest.

Spend some time massaging your man's chest, being careful not to neglect his sides, and continue pleasing his upper abdomen. Then take a comfortable position on one side to his body and continue to create good feelings in his central abdomen by playing with his belly button. Continue with his lower abdomen, but don't touch his penis or scrotum yet.

From his lower abdomen, move down and massage his hips and thighs with a combination of massage movements and a generously giving attitude. Then continue on to his knees, lower legs, feet, and toes. Move up and down from his hips to his toes a few times on each leg, switching positions to remain comfortable, going slowly and patiently without exhausting yourself.

After creating happiness in your man's legs, carefully spread his legs apart and take a kneeling position between them. Then move your palms through his thighs and up to his genitals, which are the most sensitive erogenous zone in a man's body. Dealing with your man's testicle sack and penis without developing an eager urgency in him for orgasm requires care and patience.

This is the point in amorous massage when the second magic verse must be applied without fail, although you should switch versions since the man is now on the receiving side. The woman now says, "We don't want an orgasm now," and the man says, "I don't want an orgasm now." When the woman is ready to perform amorous massage on the man's genitals, both of you must start to recite your respective versions of the second magic verse to yourselves. The first magic verse, "Making you happy makes me happy," is also important and should be active in the woman's heart since she is now in the giving role.

The woman now starts to massage her beloved man's scrotum and penis with the attitude that she really enjoys it. Starting with his testicle pouch, hold it between your hands firmly enough to create feeling. Make sure that you aren't hurting him and move slowly and carefully, but playfully enjoy yourself. Treat the penis and testicles as one piece of dough, and perform doughing with rotations and zigzags, pulling and pushing up and down as though actually conditioning the "dough." Here the third magic verse, "Slow and long," must be applied. All movements must be slow and long to make sure that you're not developing urgency for orgasm. Work on your man's testicle sack and penis in great detail, just as he did with your vagina.

The man should relish this intensely wonderful feeling, but keep chanting your version of the second magic verse so that you won't lose self-control.

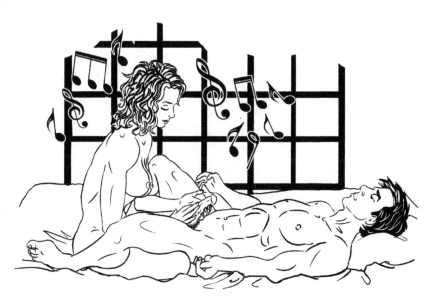

The woman continues to lovingly dough her partner's genitals with a gracious, giving attitude. After making his genitals happy for three or four minutes, smoothly slide your hand across his belly and chest to his face and bestow a passionate kiss on his lips. The man should fully give himself to that kiss and then open his eyes.

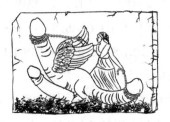

Nineteen

Extreme 69

B oth people should now be at the peak of their lust, ready to merge with the other and become a single living organism that disappears into a whirlwind of erotic bliss. The strangely interesting experience of oral sex is a good way to start, even though oral sex isn't a component of the basic sexual act. Oral sex is actually a perversion, but a positive one. At the height of sexual excitement, women and men often become greedy for even more good feeling, and that leads them to engage in oral sex. Common sense tells us that as long as the participants aren't hurting each other, there is absolutely nothing wrong with indulging in oral sex.

Humans tend to get a thrill from breaking rules and crossing lines, and this psychology might be a factor in our enjoyment of oral sex. No matter why we do it, an ultra-intimate situation is created when one person's face and mouth are interacting with the utmost private parts between the legs of another person, and vice versa. Even men and women who share no emotional bond sometimes have oral sex, but when it happens in an emotionally committed, loving relationship, oral sex has a deeper, more gratifying meaning. So it seems perfectly appropriate for it to be part of this wonderful ceremony of lovemaking.

At this point in our Hot Break, mutual oral sex play is the preferable path, which means that it's time for sex position 69 or what I like to call "Extreme 69."

After that passionate kiss at the end of the amorous massage, the man should kiss the woman's chin and shoulder, shower tongue-swirl kisses on both of her breasts, and then plant tongue-swirl kisses all the way from her belly to her lower abdomen. The woman should do the same to her partner, moving synchronously with him from his lips to his chin, shoulder, and lower abdomen, spreading tongue-swirl kisses everywhere.

The man moves from the woman's lower belly to her hips and then her inner thighs, scattering dragging-tongue-spin kisses and finally arriving at her mysterious vagina. The woman moves simultaneously from his lower belly to his hips and then his inner thighs with dragging-tongue-whirl kisses, and from there makes her way to his penis, which is probably fully erect and demanding, where she takes his scrotum in one hand.

The woman and man now lie side by side, facing each other, with their heads comfortably supported by each other's thigh and connected to each other's genitals with their mouths. This is the Extreme 69 sex position, which is actually a simultaneous combination of cunnilingus and fellatio. All movements in this position must be slow and long to avoid developing an urgency for orgasm in both of you.

At this point, the first magic verse, "Making you happy makes me happy," and the second version of the second magic verse, "We don't want an orgasm now," must be continuously active in the minds of both people. Extreme 69 is a crazy, ultra-intense sex ride and a strangely enjoyable positive perversion. You disappear between the legs of your beloved one and enjoy their genitals with licks, sucks, and tongue spins for as long as you both want, without any hurry and with extreme care for each other. Let the Extreme 69 euphoria continue for three to four minutes, while carefully remaining in full control by continuously applying the second magic verse.

Everyone's situation is different, and outward projections sometimes don't match inner reality. For people who are incapable of engaging in penetrative sex, Extreme 69 can take you all the way to the final fireworks. In that kind of situation, let the Extreme 69 celebration go on until both partners feel like they're ready for the finale, and they can stimulate each other with mouth and hands and end up in two or more fiery orgasms!

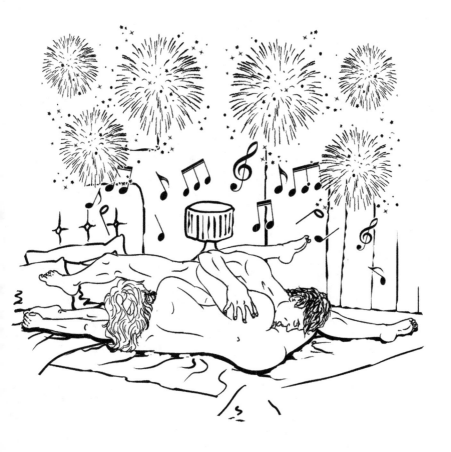

Twenty

Ultimate Embrace

I f you are not moving for the finale at this point enjoy the Extreme 69 as long as you both want to. When both of you feel like turn around and merge into a passionate embrace and kiss. You are now at the most crucial point in this amazing ceremony of lovemaking, to the intercourse stage. Don't pause and let the woody soften. Inside the ambience of soft light and romantic music, the man moves over and sits on the edge of the bed with his feet on the floor and slowly pulls his beloved woman toward him. The woman places her legs on either side of his body and sits on his lap, comfortably allowing his eagerly erect penis to enter her like silk, and they lovingly embrace.

Completely immersed in the ultimate intimate experience, enjoy the warmth and presence inside each other's arms, woman on man's lap and he is inside her and she slowly begins to rotate and thrust. There's no reason to hurry, so act with determined patience and concentrate on the exact places from which the good feeling is coming. As one variation of sitting position, this is the most affectionate and intimate condition that a man and woman can attain because an embrace is a natural part of this sex position. In this ultimate erotic hug, the man and woman actually becomes a single living organism.

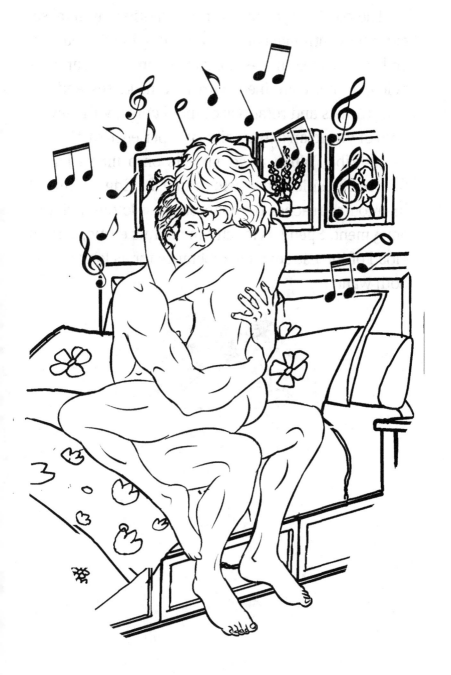

The condition of being in an emotionally intense, extremely intimate embrace and enjoying the warmth and texture of skin-to-skin connection with your most beloved one, combined with fervent kisses and the slow thrusts and rotations of intercourse, will elevate both of you to an extraordinary experience that's hard to describe. When a woman sits on a man's lap in this sex position, the astounding feeling of sexual intercourse reaches the highest, most loving point of enjoyment. Spend as much time in this erotic, surreal cloud of intense sexual exuberance for as long as you both want.

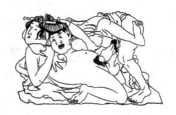

Twenty-One

Table or Wall

A man and woman engaged in an ultimate embrace can smoothly morph into another erotic position to avoid any chance of monotony. The man and woman both leave the bed and move to a wall where the woman leans back and the man kisses her fervently on the lips and both breasts, using his tongue to play with her nipples. Then, with very little pause, he lifts and holds one of her legs in a comfortable position, enters her from the front, and they begin to slowly thrust and rotate. They continue to enjoy the abundance of ecstasy for as long as they want, because there is no rush when you're on a Hot Break.

The woman also can lie back on a table, and the man stands between her legs and enters her from the front. This face-to-face act of erotic union allows the woman and man to see and enjoy the surges and waves happening to each other, which raises the acutely sweet experience of sex to unexpected levels. These frontal sex positions also give the man tempting access to the woman's breasts; he can play with them, softly squeeze them, and love her nipples with kisses, tongue swirls, and sucking. The man is now inside his woman, lovingly playing with her breasts while engaged in long, slow thrusts of passionate intercourse. The woman can keep her legs comfortably against the wall, on a chair, or on his shoulders. During intercourse, they can warmly run their hands over each other's arms, shoulders and back to further enhance the wholeness of the good feeling of lust.

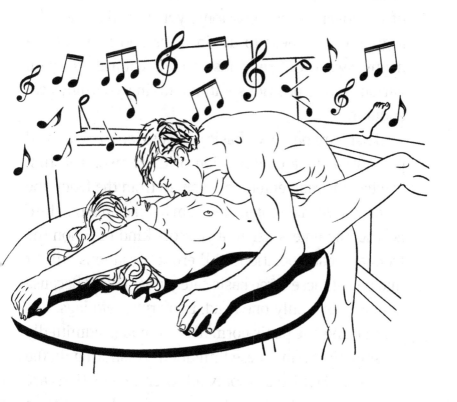

Don't forget—there's no hurry, because you're on a well-planned Hot Break. So relish the good feelings coming from every part of your bodies, particularly the erogenous zones such as the vagina, penis, breasts, and lips. Let your lovemaking continue for several minutes. At this point in the sensually charged phase of the lovemaking ceremony, you're both driven by a greedy eagerness to attain more and more of the happy, sweet torture of lust, so you can ride through various erotic positions without taxing your physical endurance.

There are only two basic sex positions, and a third position that's a combination of those two. The first is when the man enters the woman from the front, the second is when he enters her from behind, and the third is when he enters her in a scissors kind of union the front and back positions. All erotic variations will fit into one of these three basic categories. This is because humans have only one head, two arms, two legs, one vagina, and one penis normally—although admittedly we sometimes find these limitations frustrating. In the context of Hot Breaks, only a few erotic positions are considered, with the goal of improving the quality of affectionate bonding between a man and a woman with love.

You and your beloved partner are now on the table or against the wall, actively engaged in passionate intercourse, so let it continue as long as you both want.

When you agree that you both want to try another sex position, the man can smoothly separate from the woman and help her lovingly back to the bed.

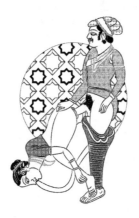

Twenty-Two

Lovingly from Behind

N ow let the heat and thrill of lust go up little more higher by changing to another naughty and engrossing coitus position, that is Man from Behind the Woman sex position. Not to allow the enthusiasm of the situation to subside do not leave a pause. Woman bend over to the bed presenting yourself lustfully for your man, man approach your beloved woman from behind and enter her romantically with affection and care.

Man entering from behind is a wonderful erotic position in many ways. In this coitus position woman is amorously at the passive side presenting herself wholly to her beloved man, to receive everything she can relish by indulging in sexual intercourse. Woman can slide into her sensuous dream world to covertly enjoy inside an intense cloud of lust.

Man from Behind the Woman coitus position offers the man to take the active part which is thrilling and engaging for him to enjoy. He has the freedom to make his beloved woman happier by rubbing her back and sides and can fondle her breasts and can play with her clitoris as well, while himself enthusiastically relishing intercourse.

At this vigorously active stage of the wonderful ceremony of lovemaking on the most important day of Hot Break, woman and man give yourselves totally and consciously to enjoy all the righteous good feelings that evolve particularly because of the distinctiveness of Man from Behind the Woman coitus position. Be reminded not to miss to use the first magic verse of Hot Break, "Making you happy makes me happy," to experience the height of sensuous sensations.

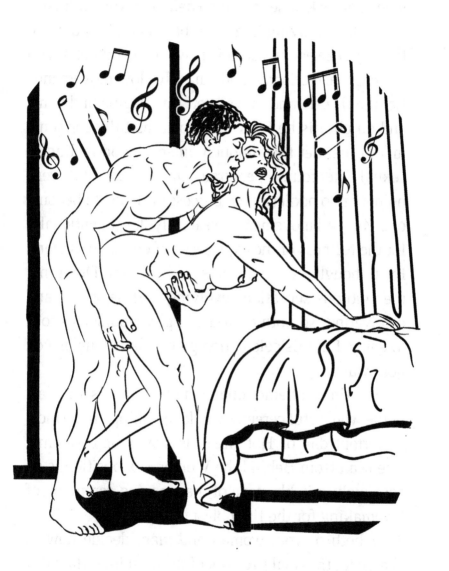

Let this joyous turmoil of sex act go on for a while. To enhance the experience of coitus, man can rub your woman's back, sides and then bent over your woman's back like an loving hug from behind and fondle and love squeeze her breasts and play with her clitoris with sincerely affectionate and caringly slow movements. Let the thrusts and moves between vagina and penis and on clitoris be Slow and Long lustfully for some more time. Let this uniquely intense good feeling of sexual intercourse penetrate and spread into every point of two bodies in the process of fusion to become one. Keep all movements sensuously slow intentionally for the fullness of the experience of erotic enjoyment. Even though the movements are Slow and Dragging, the amorous sensations evolving will be strong and captivating, so both of you can give yourselves to it to enjoy. Let this celebration go on for as long as you both want.

The finale of emotional and physical blissful blast of the wonderful ceremony of lovemaking on the most important day of Hot Break is slowly approaching. The Man from Behind the Woman sex position is an absolutely suitable stage of the amazing ceremony of lovemaking for the final blast of orgasms.

If both of you, woman and man, decide now to charge for the final firework of the most important day of Hot Break, slowly start to speed up your movements. Don't hurry, so you won't miss the romantic rhythm.

From this point onward, both of you should stop using the second and third magic verses.

Man will be the main manipulator of matters from here if you both decide to go for the final firework of the amazing ceremony of lovemaking. Woman, give your body and mind wholly to your beloved man, eagerly anticipating the final big shakeup. Man, increase the speed of intercourse movement in a steady, slow pace until you reach a continuous higher speed combining penis to vagina thrusts, caringly stimulating nipples and clitoris until the lust blast happens.

If it happens for the man first, he should not depart from the woman's vagina, but should continue stimulating her breasts and clitoris and make that big blast—the intense firework of lust and love—occur for her as well. If the woman has an orgasm first, the man can withdraw from her vagina, let her fall onto the bed and lie back flat, and, according to her comfort, continue in the classic missionary position, leading himself to the firework of a joyous erotic blast and then falling slowly onto the bed beside his beloved woman.

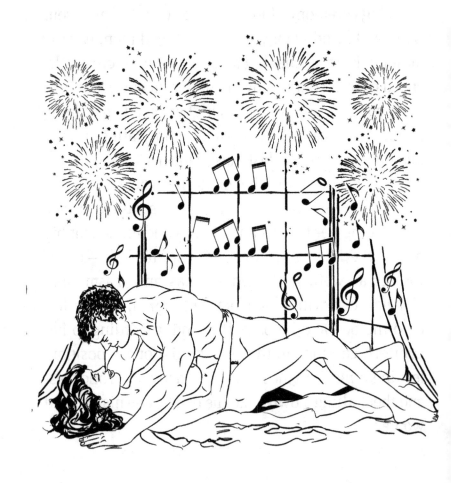

Chapter

Twenty-Three

The Finale

I f both woman and man want to take this wonderful ceremony of lovemaking a little further, the man can smoothly and slowly withdraw from Man from Behind the Woman position, lie back on the bed, and present the erect penis straight upward for his beloved woman. Without pausing, the woman can crawl toward her beloved man and romantically go over him, spreading her legs, knees on either side of his hips. In this pleasing ambience of sweet music and sizzling lust, the woman can guide her man's hard penis to slide into her smoothly. Woman is now the primary manipulator of intercourse action. Man, give yourself totally to your woman, supporting her with secondary intercourse movements. Now again, both of you can make use of the "We don't want an orgasm now" version of the second magic verse of Hot Break to extend the bliss of the wonderful ceremony of lovemaking a little longer. Woman, use slow, long thrusts and rotate in total control. Man, accompany her with the same kind of slow, long upward thrusts, playing with and sucking her breasts and engaging in deep kisses now and then as well. In this vibrancy of sex, both of you should keep your minds sharply on where the action takes place in your body and consciously relish all the intense good feeling that is evolving. Do not miss a bit of it. Be in this celebration of lust and love as long as you two want; let it go on for a while.

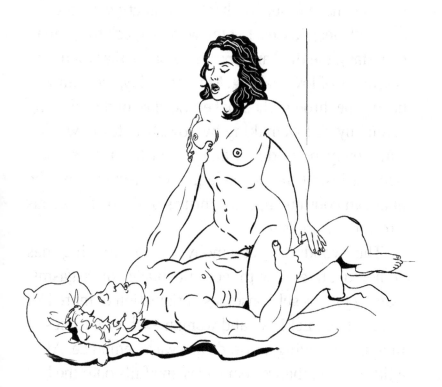

Now you two are at the most ideal point to move toward the finale of the wonderful ceremony of lovemaking. Enjoy the Woman Riding the Man erotic position for a while. If you decide to take action for the finale, you can speed up your intercourse movements slowly, rhythmically, and romantically. Let the woman lead and the man support her by stimulating her breasts and with deep kisses. Let the woman reach the climax of ecstasy, the final amorous firework of the wonderful ceremony of lovemaking. Most probably, the man will have gone through the final erotic blast of the amazing ceremony of lovemaking by now. If not, the woman can slowly bend down and lie on her man's chest without losing the penis-vagina connection, and the man can continue upward thrusts until the rapturous firework of orgasm.

The wonderful ceremony of lovemaking has come to an end with ecstatic blasts of orgasms, leaving joyous subconscious anticipation of more Hot Breaks to come! Man and woman exchange kisses of indefinable loving gratitude in a warm embrace. After a little while, the woman slides and falls onto the bed beside her beloved man, and both lie down. Now the heat of sex subsides, but the warmth of love prevails and fills the space!

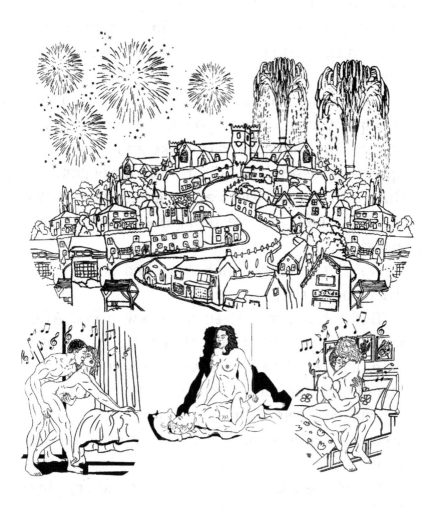

Both of you are now in bed almost totally exhausted. Do not try to hold yourselves mentally for anything. Give yourselves fully to the bed. Most probably you two will disappear into a snuggly, engulfing, one-of-a-kind sleep soon. Before sinking into that mesmerizing sleep, man, turn to your beloved woman and embrace her—maybe a half embrace, since you're in bed—and shower her with kisses on the forehead, cheeks, and lips. Woman, embrace your beloved man and gift him lavishly with kisses on the forehead, cheeks, and lips. These kisses show a distinctive kind of gratitude filled with love and happiness for granting each other the opportunity to ride through an intense, good experience.

Now let yourselves sink down and dissolve into that amorous sleep.

Both of you may sleep for a few hours. After waking up, get out of bed, each at his or her own pace, leisurely take a lukewarm shower, and dress according to the place and time of the year. Then go out into the streets and have a nice rich lunch or dinner accompanied by some wine, beer, or whatever you each like.

Spend the whole evening relaxed and enjoying. Walk around, and when it darkens, go to a bar, have a few drinks with snacks, and enjoy the ambience, possibly with music and dancing. Finally, when both of you feel like it, return to your cozy room and fall onto the bed. After some kisses and embraces, the intoxicating glee of love will naturally submerge you into a good night's sleep.

Twenty-Four

Craving More

The next morning, you two may decide to have one more most important day of Hot Break. That is absolutely a desirable and justifiable craving, so go for it. The second most important day of Hot Break will give you a chance to correct the misses that happened the first time and to add some new ideas that you got later to heighten the experience of the amazing ceremony of lovemaking. But the second most important day of Hot Break cannot be this third day of Hot Break. There should be at least a one-day gap between two most important days of Hot Break.

So spend this whole day sitting in a beautiful place and peacefully enjoying the happiness of relaxing. You can also use this day for sightseeing, eating, drinking, and sleeping.

When you wake up the next morning, start with a lukewarm shower and a nice breakfast. On the second most important day of Hot Break, do everything the same as the first most important day of Hot Break from start to finish, with improvements and additions. That will most probably take both of you through some unforeseen good experiences.

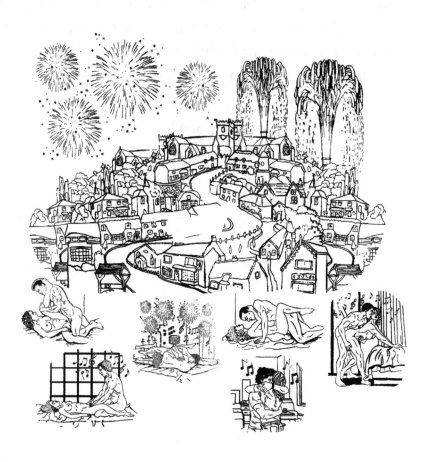

Now the time has come for man and woman to return to their real world from the wonderful world of Hot Break. You have been hallowed by the magic of Eros. The wonderful world of Hot Break is always within reach of woman and man, who can go there now and then to get rejuvenated. Man and woman, go back to your day-to-day life happily anticipating the Hot Breaks that are going to happen in the future!

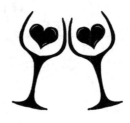

Twenty-Five

Evaluation

After those exceptional days of celebration of lust and love, man and woman may evaluate the experience they had on the most important day of Hot Break. Expectations set were romantically high, and both of you surely went through several extremely intense, good experiences of lust in the presence of love. But you may also have experienced traces of disappointment about something missed at some points in Hot Break, which is natural and realistic.

The misses in the wonderful ceremony of lovemaking might have been some unexpected pauses and loss of rhythm here and there. The man may have experienced ups and downs in penis erection, or lost control and ejaculated at an odd point. Perhaps the woman could not reach orgasm, or some totally unforeseeable things interrupted you. Keep in mind that those kinds of occurrences are not going to intercept every most important day of Hot Break for sure. Do not allow yourselves to slip into disappointment. Instead give your full attention to reminiscing and relishing all the good you experienced during Hot Break. You two can discuss even the minute details about the good things you each experienced, to enjoy the ripple effect again and again. Even if you had some disappointments, there is no reason to worry, because Hot Break is not just a one-time event. Many more Hot Breaks are in front of you, so you can reclaim what you missed in this one.

Also, if you decide to celebrate one more most important day of Hot Break during this Hot Break, right there is a chance to regain the misses. And console yourselves that during future Hot Breaks, both of you will surely improve and will be showered with more and more precious moments of lust and love.

It is a fact that Hot Breaks are not possible every day or every other day. Hot Breaks are special and should be celebrated two or three—at maximum four—times a year, not more than that. Although that may reduce the chances to correct misses, it affirms that you two should forget and leave behind the misses and should concentrate on all the good things that happened that day. You can enjoy the memories of those good things in your own private thoughts and in the secluded moments with your beloved partner to make your mundane days much more livable.

You can always look keenly for a windfall of some private time in your everyday life in your own home to celebrate a short version of the most important day of Hot Break, a quickie Hot Break. It can happen, and sometimes those will turn out to be some of the most memorable moments of your life.

A Hot Break has become a reality now, giving you wonderful experiences that will leave you and your partner with vibrant, alive diamonds and pearls of memories to look at occasionally and relish in. These diamonds and pearls accumulate from many Hot Breaks can become a joyous treasure for you two to relish as long as you both live.

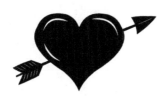

Twenty-Six

Lust Turned Love

The things that happened throughout Hot Break and especially on the most important day of Hot Break were a passage through vibrant sexual intercourse to the special place of love. When man and woman simply give their mind and body to each other, they are rewarded with the most intense ecstatic experience of life. When woman and man come together, fascinated with each other, simply because they like each other and are involved in extreme physical intimacy, nothing else really matters. Money or any other issues cannot obstruct the path to pure happiness.

When every piece of clothing falls to the floor, along with all the ego and pride, all the inhibitions between man and woman will also wither away into air. It is an amazing experience of freedom, joy, and emancipation of minds from the strain of holding so many things that are trying to separate woman and man. It is a journey of extreme physical intimacy to attain the place where there is always the spring of love. That spring will bloom now and then in Hot Breaks, and again and again in the memories of woman and man to make them love each other forever.

When every human being in this world really realizes, understands, and accepts love in all its dimensions and sincerely learns to practice it in everything of everyday life, we will find that it is the only way to achieve real happiness and make living worthwhile. In the matter of love in the relationship of man and woman, passionate sexual intercourse plays a major role in attaining that happiness.

We ride through the valley,
tremulous, warm, and cuddly,
The shimmering light of love,
which doesn't make any shadows,
shines upon our souls.

Printed in the United States
By Bookmasters